TENNIS:
Winning the Mental Game

D1594368

Robert Weinberg, Ph.D.

Miami University

Oxford, Ohio

Acknowledgments

As is typically the case, this book would not have been possible if not for the help of many people. I will try to acknowledge these important individuals, but if I miss someone, it's only because my memory has let me down. First, let me give a big thanks to the staff at H.O. Zimman, Inc. for helping make this book possible. In particular, special thanks to Cheryl Lampert for the excellent design of the cover, and Susan Macdonald, Ericka Benham and Stefanie Pinette for the layout. But most of all a great big thanks to Adam Scharff, who helped me through every aspect of the book and provided sage guidance and advice in making the many decisions necessary to bring the book to fruition.

Second, I'd like to thank the following people for either posing for, or being in the photographs inside the book: Ken Alrutz, Erica Echko, Champy Halim, Amin Nabli, Kadija Richards, and Ray Reppert. Third, I'd like to thank my many sport psychology and tennis colleagues who offered advice and feedback on different aspects of the book, as well as providing some of the research and practice upon which this book was based. Thanks to all the individuals who read through the book prior to publication and offered feedback regarding the content of the book. In particular, a big thanks to Ray Reppert, whose tennis expertise and enthusiasm for the project helped me immeasurably.

Finally, let me also thank my wife, Cynthia Goodman, for reading the book and providing feedback from proofreading to content to presentation. This helped make the book read and look a great deal better. She deserves a great deal of thanks for her patience in allowing me the time and space needed to write this book. Her unconditional social support was always there just when I needed it. So a big thanks.

Dedication

To my family, the most important part of my life.

Front Cover Photography: Ron Angle (Agassi); Andy Jacobs (Capriati).
Photography: Jeffrey Sabo (Back Cover, Chapter 3 and Chapters 5-11).

Produced by H.●. ZIMMAN, Inc.

ISBN-0-972-0940-0-8

Contents

Foreword

Having been involved in the world of tennis for many years as a player, coach, and owner, I have seen all styles of play and many different types of competitors. What always amazed me was not only the different physical abilities and strokes players brought to the court, but also the various attitudes and mental approaches players possessed. There are players of all levels of ability who just can't seem to win matches, even though they have beautiful, well-manicured strokes, obviously developed under the careful scrutiny of a tennis pro. And then there are those who don't have classic strokes or a lot of natural stroking ability, but somehow know how to win. In watching the latter type of player play over the years, it became abundantly clear to me that there is something more to winning than just possessing proficient strokes (although that is a good start). Nice strokes can be learned simply by following the instructions given by a good coach or teaching pro. Repetition will usually suffice to bring your shot-making abilities to a reasonable level. But how to use these skills more effectively is much more difficult and complicated. Here, strategy, knowledge of the game, and mental skills become very important.

This is where Weinberg's book comes into play. It is a serious, thoughtful, and research-based approach to the mental side of tennis, and it will help you take stock of your game. Although many players and coaches have made references to the importance of mental skills (especially when tennis players are of reasonably similar ability), few have really tried to practice these skills in any sort of systematic fashion. Part of the reason is that most coaches and teaching pros don't know how to specifically work on mental skills, such as coping with anxiety, improving concentration, enhancing confidence, and sustaining motivation. It is this need that prompted Weinberg to write this practical guide for tennis players, teachers, and coaches. His expertise in sport psychology as well as experiences as a tennis coach and player has helped him write a hands-on book, filled with exercises, tips, and strategies that are easily understandable by tennis players of all ages and abilities.

Weinberg captures the reader's attention with his insightful writing and the manner in which he utilizes quotes, anecdotes, and examples from high visibility professional players, as well as more recreational players, to bring to life some of the key points. He emphasizes the importance of developing and practicing mental skills, highlighting the mental skills that are integral for peak performance on the tennis court and then providing specific ways to practice and achieve these optimal conditions.

The chapters on mental preparation and the psychology of match play are especially meaningful and important to me. They are two areas I emphasized a great deal during my own days as a professional. Certainly, playing Bobby Riggs in front of a huge TV audience required lots of mental preparation and the ability to deal with gamesmanship. But then again, so did playing in Grand Slams and other tennis matches. Another area that is not stressed enough, which Weinberg so deftly points out, is communication between doubles partners. The practical tips he provides should go a long way in helping players fine-tune their games.

So whether you're a professional player or a recreational one, don't underestimate the mental side of the game. If you are already a serious tennis player, or if you want to be, then this book offers many challenges and ways to achieve them. It's often easier to see the physical aspect of the game, but don't be fooled. It's really what's between the ears that really counts. I've played against both types, and believe me, players who have their mental game together, are always harder to beat. Weinberg has now given you an easy way to understand, develop, and practice these mental skills. So now it's up to you to. Go for it.

Billie Jean King

Preface

Most competitive tennis players spend many hours each week, training physically and technically to enhance their games. There are all sorts of rallying, conditioning, and footwork drills that help players master these fundamental skills. There is nothing wrong with this approach. In fact, it is quite essential when learning the game of tennis to understand and master the basic skills and strategies involved. But we all know that winning tennis matches goes far beyond strokes and techniques. This idea is highlighted by Brad Gilbert's (1993) book entitled *Winning Ugly*. Although Brad Gilbert (who also was Andre Agassi's coach for many years) was not one of the most talented professional tennis players and did not possess classic strokes, he rose to be one of the top ten players in the world. He accomplished this amazing feat by spending lots of attention on the mental aspects of tennis and focusing on winning the mental game (since he couldn't always win the physical game).

In doing workshops with tennis players and coaches, I usually ask them how important is the mental aspect of tennis (as compared to the physical) when it comes to being successful and winning matches? The typical response is that it is very important and becomes more and more important as the level and ability of the tennis players increase. Yet most players and coaches readily admit that they spend very little time on the mental aspects of tennis (although this has been improving over the past 10 years). This is most often due to the fact that coaches and tennis pros do not know how to teach mental skills like improving concentration, managing anxiety and building confidence (however, in recent years most coaches and players seem eager to learn about developing these mental skills as sport psychology has become more popular).

As a result, most tennis books, instructional camps, teaching pros, and coaches emphasize the physical side of tennis. There is a wealth of information out there in tennis books and magazines, if you want to learn about weight transfer, body mechanics, footwork, topspins, stroke production, racquet angles, string tensions, etc. It is nice to see that *Tennis Magazine* now routinely has a brief column called "The Mental Notebook" which is devoted to the mental aspects of tennis. Obviously, people in the tennis world are realizing the critical role the mind plays in reaching one's potential as a tennis player (or maybe they knew about it for awhile but now they are writing about it). In fact, the United States Tennis Association has developed a set of player competencies that includes a section on the mental aspects of tennis as well as a coaches' guide to sport psychology. This underscores the central role that psychology plays in developing young tennis players.

When I published *The Mental Advantage: Developing Your Psychological Skills in Tennis* in 1988, we were just starting to get an understanding of the mental side of tennis. However, over the past 15 years, sport psychologists have made major strides in developing mental and psychological strategies to help enhance the performance and personal growth of performers in a wide variety of sports. We have a much better understanding of how to train tennis players from a mental perspective and the principles of mental training have been developed through careful and systematic on-court work with tennis players and coaches. But what has remained constant, or has become even more apparent, is how important mental training is to the development of current tennis players. To highlight this point, I was recently asked to present a keynote talk to the British Association for Sport and Exercise on "Developing the Perfect Tennis Player: Emphasis on the Mental Perspective" (maybe they are looking for an English Wimbledon champion).

Along these lines, the crucial role that the mind plays in competitive tennis has become clearer and clearer to me over the years through my roles and experience as a tennis player, coach, and sport psychologist, consulting with tennis players. For example, in observing and playing in many tennis matches, I began to realize that the player with the better strokes, footwork, form, and coordination did not necessarily win the match (Brad Gilbert highlighted this point). Players with superior skills would invariably walk off the tennis court in disbelief mumbling to themselves, "How could she possibly beat me? She doesn't have any strokes?" But that is just the point. Nice strokes do not necessarily win competitive tennis matches; it takes a total effort and commitment to endure highly competitive tennis matches. Brad Gilbert is a perfect example of this concept.

To give a personal example, I grew up in New York City playing mostly team sports (e.g., basketball, football, baseball). There were not even places to play tennis in my neighborhood and moreover, tennis was considered a "sissy sport." But one summer at camp as a counselor, I learned to play tennis (about age 19) but I never took any formal lessons. Rather, I relied on my athletic ability and mental toughness learned from my experience in team sports to transfer to my tennis game. As a result, I have never developed what you would call classical strokes. Yet, I have competed fairly successfully at the collegiate and senior levels, relying heavily on my mental game, rather than my physical game (in retrospect it seems too bad that my mental game really started to get strong just at the time my physical prowess was starting to show signs of aging). In fact, I would probably be one of those players you might be infuriated to lose to because I do not possess particularly good strokes.

But this mental struggle described above is not necessarily against an opponent. Rather, it is a struggle that goes on inside ourselves; a struggle to win the mental game. Because if we can win the mental game, we probably will not only perform better, but (and probably more importantly) the game itself will be more fun and enjoyable. It is my belief that most competitive tennis players and coaches are eager to learn more about how to develop this elusive mental game. This need and interest convinced me of the necessity of trying to update my original work so that I could provide coaches and players with more cutting-edge material on mental training techniques. Along these lines, sport psychology has developed considerably and we now know a great deal more about mental training and the techniques that form the backbone of this training. In addition, similar to my first book, I believe that an action-oriented approach should be taken highlighting specific exercises, strategies, and techniques that players and coaches could use and incorporate into their regular practices. That is, a research-to-practice orientation will be followed attempting to translate the most current sport psychology knowledge to enhancing your mental skills in tennis. In summary, the major objectives of the book are as follows:

(a) To highlight the importance of the mental side of tennis to players and coaches and demonstrate that these mental skills can be taught and need to be practiced.

(b) To describe the psychological states that are associated with peak performance and how to enhance the occurrence of these states.

(c) To discuss the importance of motivation and commitment to implementing a mental training program.

(d) To provide a background as to why and how specific mental skills (e.g., self-talk, goal-setting, anxiety management, imagery) can help players reach their full potentials.

(e) To detail specific techniques, exercises, and programs to practice developing these skills

(f) To demonstrate that these mental skills in tennis can not only enhance performance, but can also lead to greater enjoyment and fun participating in sport.

CHAPTER 1

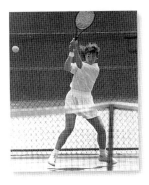

THE MENTAL SIDE OF TENNIS: WHY IS IT SO IMPORTANT?

Have you ever walked off tennis court in disgust because you lost a match you felt you should have won? Have you ever lacked the commitment or desire to "hang in" a long tough match or practice consistently? Has your mind ever wandered during a match to think about other things or possibly a previous point? Have you ever gotten tight and maybe even "choked" at a critical point in a match? Have you ever become frustrated and angry during a match, calling yourself names or maybe even throwing the racquet? Have you ever gotten upset or lost your cool after getting a bad line call? Have you ever let the antics of an opponent "get to you" and cause you to lose your concentration?

If you answered yes to any of these questions, don't feel bad because you have a lot of company. In fact, as a player, coach, and sport psychologist, it has been my experience that it would be extremely rare (if not impossible) to find a tennis player who has not suffered through one or more of the above scenarios. Nobody who has played tennis with any intensity or passion would dispute the statement that beyond the purely physical and technical aspects of the game, is a mental or emotional component that often overshadows or transcends the physical aspects. All of us know what it feels like to be "in the zone" where everything seems to be flowing and winners fly effortlessly off our racquets (even if this feeling is infrequent). Conversely, we all have had days when nothing seemed to go right, we felt tight and uncomfortable, and every shot was an adventure. Through the exercises and knowledge you hopefully will gain from this book, it is my firm belief that you can make it more probable that you will get into flow more often and thus enjoy your tennis more.

Why is Tennis Difficult From a Mental Standpoint?

If you stand and watch recreational or competitive players play for awhile, you will inevitably see or hear emotional outbursts, swearing, people talking to themselves, and possibly some ball or racquet abuse. These people are, by and large, rational, controlled people away from the game of tennis. So what is it about tennis that makes it so difficult from a mental perspective? First of all, tennis is a very exacting game requiring a precise combination of timing, coordination, decision-making, quickness, focused attention, and stamina. But let's focus for a moment on the decision-making aspect. For example, it has been found that in the average tennis match, approximately 800-1,200 decisions have to be made, with most of these having to be made in less than one second. If you decide to play conservatively, just keeping the ball in play, and your opponent takes the offensive and hits a winner, you will probably be mad that you didn't make the decision to hit out and play more aggressively. But if you decide to hit out, playing more aggressively, and over-hit the ball, then you have to make an initial decision and you often can be caught second-guessing yourself wondering why you didn't play more conservatively.

Second, from a biomechanical point of view, if your racquet face varies by just a couple of degrees, this will likely result in hitting the ball into the bottom of the net or way past the baseline. Thus, being able to repeatedly and consistently find the exact racquet angle for different shots can be very frustrating. Third, and maybe most importantly, the stop and go nature of tennis distinguishes it from many sports that are basically continuous in nature such as basketball, soccer, and hockey. In essence, tennis presents the mind with lots of "dead time" (especially between points and on changeovers), and this places great stress on the mind. In fact, in a typical tennis match, it has been found that one-quarter of the time is actually spent playing tennis with the other three-quarters being spent between points and during changeovers. So in a two hour match, you are probably only actually playing tennis about 30 minutes. During this "dead time" the mind is likely to wander and often gets absorbed in many other distractions ranging from "I hope I don't double fault and choke on my second serve" to " I have a big business meeting tomorrow that I have to be ready for." But even during the points, especially on slower surfaces like clay, the game becomes a mental battle as points are longer and more and more decisions have to be made. There is often time enough between shots to have to make decisions about shot selection and this can most definitely weigh on a player's mind. In essence, tennis often forces the mind to make abrupt switches from thought to action and this invariably produces mental errors which in turn can produce technical errors in stroke production.

This excess "thinking time" is what makes golf such a difficult game (beyond the precision needed to execute successful swings) as there is lots of time between shots. You might think this is a good thing, but, unfortunately, most people think about the wrong things during this time and often get too nervous thinking too much. This is seen in basketball where it is typical for a coach to call time-out when an opposing player is about to shoot critical free-throws at the end of a game. The reason is to give the player plenty of time to think about the importance of the shot and hopefully tighten up. In fact, this is usually called "freezing the shooter." Turning back to tennis, in my playing, coaching, and counseling experience with tennis players, most agree that the two toughest shots to hit from a mental standpoint are the serve and overhead smash. Although these two shots are certainly difficult from a technical standpoint, what makes them particularly hard is that the player usually has time to think before hitting each shot, This thinking time allows distractions and irrelevant thoughts to enter the mind, thereby disrupting timing and coordination.

There are several other things that make tennis especially tough from a mental perspective, including the following:

(a) *Calling of lines.* This is one of the few sports that during competition you have to act as referee as well as player. Tempers can flare, conflicts can arise, and this adds to the mental aspect of the game;

(b) *No substitutes or time-outs.* Play is continuous and you can't get the help of a break in the action;

(c) *Nowhere to hide.* As an individual sport you are out in the open for everyone to see every little (or not so little) mistake which can cause embarrassment, discouragement, or anger;

(d) *No coaching,* Coaching is not allowed in most situations so you're on your own to figure things out; and

(e) *Scoring system.* First, one is never going to lose a tennis match due to time running out. So even if you are way behind, you can always come back, which keeps the final outcome uncertain. In a USTA match I played a few years ago, I split sets and was down 5-0, 40-15 in the third and final set and was just hoping to get a game. But I managed to hang in there and win one game at a time and eventually the third set 7-5 (after having 8 match points against me). Time never ran out. The main point of all of this is that tennis puts great pressure on the mind from a variety of perspectives and we have to somehow turn this into executing the proper shots, at the proper time, properly. The key, therefore, is to develop a better understanding of how the body and mind can work together.

Relationship Between the Body and Mind

Since the mid 1970s, there has been a growing body of scientific evidence emphasizing the integration of body and mind. The key point research has revealed, is that our mental state can have an important impact on our physiological systems, even those we thought were more automatic in nature. Specifically, our state of mind can impact our autonomic nervous system reactions such as heart rate, respiration rate, muscle tension, and galvanic skin response (i.e., sweating) which in the past was believed to be out of our control. For example, with proper training, most of us can be taught to reduce tension in specific muscles in the body or to slow down our heart rates when we're getting too nervous. In addition, we see the body-mind relationship at work with the research indicating that athletes with high levels of anxiety are more likely to become injured. Similarly, the best predictor of your recuperation from surgery is your mental attitude. Finally, individuals with good imagery skills heal faster from injury than those who have poorer imagery skills. Thus, what we think about and how we think, most certainly can influence how our body reacts.

The Mental Side of Tennis

So, how important are these mental skills for tennis players? It is difficult to get an exact scientific answer to this question, but some anecdotal data would indicate it is very important. More specifically, I have asked tennis coaches and players, "How important are the mental and physical capabilities of a tennis player for determining success?" To answer this question, I typically ask both coaches and players in my workshops to rate the importance of the mental and physical side of tennis. By their own admission, almost all coaches and players felt that tennis success (i.e., performing up to one's capabilities) was at least 50% mental, with many indicating that it was 80% to 90% mental. These percentages held true regardless of age, gender, or ability of the players in my informal survey conducted over the past 5 years. Similarly, in past interviews, Jimmy Connors has stated that he felt tennis was 95% mental at the professional level and of course, Connors was especially known for his mental tenacity and toughness. Finally, when Eliot Teltscher, USTA National Coach and former coach of up-and-coming Taylor Dent, was asked about his pupil he replied, *His physical game is sometimes ahead of his mental game. He's now trying to figure out how to set up and play points.. He's got the physical tools, but now he's got to figure out where to hit it* (part of the decision-making noted earlier—*USTA Magazine,* 2001, p.16).

Another way to look at the importance of the mental side of tennis is to compare two of the greatest women tennis players of all time—Chris Evert and Martina Navratilova. Evert was never known as a particularly great athlete, yet she was ranked number 1 in the world for many years and has achieved a record of consistency that has been unsurpassed in recent years. When she played, the consensus among the players was that nobody was better mentally. Her concentration has been said to be unwavering regardless of line calls, distractions, or opponent's antics. Conversely, Martina Navratilova was known for her athleticism including strength, speed, quickness, and superb shot-making. Yet for several years she continually came up short in the big matches and would make critical mistakes at inappropriate times. But to her credit, Martina worked hard on the mental side of her game and became ranked number 1 in the world with an incredible string of consecutive victories. The rivalry that developed between Martina and Chris became one of the best of all time.

More recently, Martina Hingis and Serena and Venus Williams provide similar examples. Hingis had been ranked number 1 in the world for several years, mostly due to her uncanny ability to hit the right shot at the right time. She doesn't hit the ball as hard as some other top players but her mental game has always been extremely strong. Conversely, Venus and Serena Williams bring unparalleled athleticism to tennis but had some trouble early in their careers choosing the proper shots for the proper times as well as maintaining a steady, consistent level of play. But in recent years, their mental game has gotten much stronger as they have won Grand Slam tournaments and are generally much more consistent in their play. Finally, there is Jennifer Capriati, who mentally was down and out for several years (in fact was out of tennis for several years), although she was always known as someone with great strokes and physical ability. When she finally dedicated herself (both physically and mentally) she came back and eventually won several Grand Slam tournaments and became one of the top players in the game.

What Mental Skills Should be Taught

So if you buy the argument that mental skills are important for tennis success, then what techniques should be taught? Researchers (Gould, Medbery, Damarjian, & Lauer, 1999) asked just this question to coaches of 12, 14, and 16 and under players. Results were fairly consistent across age groups although there were some differences (see Table 1.1). First, the two most consistent mental skills noted by coaches were enjoyment/fun and focus/concentration. The focus on enjoyment is consistent with recent goal-setting research (Weinberg Burton, Yukelson, & Weigand, 1993; 2000) which has found that colle-

Table 1.1	The Three Most Important Mental Skills Needed By Junior Tennis Age Groups				

12 and under		14 and under		16 and under	
Enjoyment/fun	27.3%	Enjoyment/fun	14.3%	Focus/concentration	12.1%
Focus/concentration	10.0%	Focus/concentration	10.0%	Enjoyment/fun	10.8%
Emotional control	8.2%	Goal setting	9.7%	Motivation/passion	8.4%
Honesty-integrity	8.2%	Self-confidence	8.4%	Goal setting	8.0%
Self-confidence	7.8%	Motivation/passion	7.8%	Practice intensity	6.7%
Motivation/passion	7.8%	Emotional control	7.8%	Self-confidence	6.3%
Keeping competition in perspective	6.9%	Practice intensity	6.7%	Emotional control	6.1%
Positive thinking/ self-talk	5.6%	Positive thinking/ self-talk	6.1%	Personal responsibility	5.4%
Goal setting	5.4%				

Note: Mental skills given by respondents greater than 5% of the time are in the table.

giate and Olympic athletes view enjoyment/fun as one of their top three goals. Thus, even with the pressure of winning and performing well at the top levels, athletes are still reporting that having fun is a critical element in staying with the sport and keeping motivated. You will see that one's goals in tennis will have an important influence on enjoyment levels. Furthermore, presented later in the book will be research on burnout of young tennis players, and we will see that lack of fun and motivation are prime determinants for leaving the sport.

The importance of focus and concentration is to be expected as players often refer to losing or maintaining concentration as being instrumental to their failure or success. We will discuss ways to enhance concentration later in the book. Some interesting differences did arise relating to the use of goal setting and emotional control. Specifically, for the younger players (12 and under) emotional control was seen as a top priority whereas goal setting was near the bottom of the list. Conversely, for the older players (under 16), goal setting was seen as being very important with emotional control down on the list. These findings could be attributed to developmental differences, which should always be an important consideration for any tennis coach (some developmental differences are discussed in Chapter 12).

How Much Time Do You Spend Practicing the Mental Side of Tennis?

Besides asking about the importance of the mental side of tennis, I also ask workshop participants, "How much time do you usually spend mentally and physically practicing in a typical week?" Their responses reveal that most competitive tennis players spend 10-20 hours per week physically practicing (this figure is lower for the typical club player). But when asked about their mental game, most players respond that they practice mentally very little, usually just getting mentally ready for a match. However, I should note that both coaches and players have been getting better in recent years in incorporating mental practice into physical practice, as the importance of the mental game is realized.

The interesting thing is that when most players come off the court after a loss or simply not playing well, they tend to attribute their loss or poor play to psychological factors such as, "I just couldn't concentrate," "I got too tight on the important points," "I just didn't have any confidence in my strokes today," or "I just wasn't up for the match today." These attributions to mental factors being responsible for a loss is even more typical when we play against someone who has reasonably equal physical abilities (isn't that the aim of most leagues and programs—to match players of similar ability). Although certain players are known for exceptional physical ability or a particular shot—Pete Sampras (serve), Patrick Rafter (volley), Martina Hingis (movement), Andre Agassi (return of serve), Gustavo Kuerten (backhand), Lindsay Davenport (forehand)—in general, there is not a lot of difference in players in terms of their physical abilities. In fact, the outcome of many matches is typically determined by the outcome of a few critical points. Interestingly, at times in a close match, the player who wins fewer points can actually win the match, if the points she wins are the critical ones. So winning break points, or in general, taking advantage of your opportunities when given them, is often the key to success (see Chapter 12 for a discussion of one type of critical points, set-up points). For example, in a recent Wimbledon match, Goran Ivanisevic served approximately 50 aces against Yevgeny Kafelnikov but still lost the match. Kafelnikov had to be patient to take his opportunities when they came his way.

The ideas presented above do not just pertain to professional players. At all levels of play, people are generally matched according to ability and thus "A" players play "A" players and players rated at 4.5 tend to play other 4.5 players. Thus, in most of your matches, you probably have a reasonable chance of either winning or losing, depending upon how you play that particular day. So some days you can defeat an opponent 6-2, 6-3, but play that player a week later and you can lose 6-2, 6-3. Did your physical ability change so much in a week's time? Not likely. But what is more likely is that your mental game has fluctuated greatly causing a very different outcome.

Why is the Mental Side Not Practiced

If both coaches and players agree that the mental side of tennis is critical to becoming a successful player, then why is so little time and emphasis generally put on practicing or developing one's mental skills? From talking to coaches as well as some recent research with coaches (Gould, Guinan, Greenleaf, Medberry & Peterson, 1999; Gould et al.,1999) there appear to be a number of reasons why these skills are either not practiced at all or given superficial attention. We will focus on some of the more major issues cited by coaches.

Lack of Coaching Education

The reason most often provided by coaches as to why they don't teach mental skills is that there has been a lack of coaching education specific to teaching these skills. Three related themes fitting under the general dimension of coaching education include (a) not knowing the process of teaching mental skills; (b) not understanding mental skills training content; and (c) not knowing alternative mediums for conveying mental skills training information. As one coach said, "I think there still needs to be more information, more feedback, so that we can get more tapes and more books." Another coach thinks that books are not enough saying, "You can read a book or an article, but does the tennis pro know how to take that book and translate it to on-court experience for the kids to learn?"

Coaches have been known to just tell players "to concentrate" or "just relax" but these instructions carry no information about how to accomplish increased concentration or relaxation. You would not be expected to execute, for example, a difficult half-volley if you had not practiced this shot again and again. So how is a player going to concentrate or relax (particularly at the most difficult and pressure-filled times) if she has not been taught and practiced these skills? Fortunately, I have noticed that more and more coaches are getting some training or taking some courses in sport psychology and mental skill training to help learn about how to teach these skills. As noted earlier, the USTA has included a section on sport psychology in their training of coaches as one example of its increased visibility. However, few coaches appear to actually implement any formal, systematic mental training program with their tennis players. In essence, there is usually only "lip service" paid to the importance of the mental side, both from coaches and players alike.

Lack of Comfort Teaching Mental Skills

A lot of the above hesitancy in teaching mental skills all boils down to one's comfort level in teaching these specific skills. As one coach said, "I did a lot more mental stuff the last year and a half or 2 years. I was slow getting into it simply because it's out of my comfort zone... It is different from teaching a forehand or serve." Another coach expresses the same feeling about comfort saying, "I think that you have to be taught how to teach mental skills...If you're not comfortable with it yourself, you're not going to relate it real well to the kids. So the information is there, but I think it has to be taught to the coaches a little better so they're comfortable with it."

Other Roadblocks to Teaching Mental Skills

There are a number of other important reasons why coaches don't systematically teach mental skills including the following:

- Lack of Time—Although this is usually more perceived lack of time than actual lack of time;
- Lack of Interest on Part of the Players—This should not be a problem as many examples of top players can be used to motivate lesser players. The problem might be in devising interesting drills to practice mental training;
- Difficult to Evaluate Mental Training Success—It is always more difficult to evaluate the effect of mental training than physical training, but there are ways to do this (I will provide some examples in the upcoming chapters).

How to Make Mental Skill Training More User-Friendly

So if coaches and players feel that mental skills are important, how can the teaching of these skills be made more user-friendly, so that coaches can teach, and players can learn these valuable mental skills? Again, research with tennis pros and coaches gives us some good suggestions to follow and I will highlight two of these:

- Make mental skills more concrete. As one tennis coach noted, "I like examples— examples of what happened, what you are thinking, and what is going on. If you came up with a book of examples of players, that would be an easy way to get started."
- Provide various mediums for coaches and players. Use of videotape, CDs, computer

games and computer web-sites were mentioned as possibilities. More specifically, a video showing coaches giving mental skills talks and leading exercises as well as a CD-ROM or computer disc explaining mental skills, drills and exercises were two suggestions. As a coach noted, "I think through pictures; I think that shows a lot. Just what a mentally tough competitor looks like, depending on whether they are winning or losing."

Mental Skills Can Be Learned if Practiced Regularly

The above discussion leads us to one of the major purposes of this book; that is, to provide tennis players and coaches who are serious about improving their games, with specific ideas, techniques, exercises, and strategies concerning the mental aspects of tennis. I will try to demonstrate that certain mental states are consistently associated with higher levels of tennis performance. Consistently achieving these mental states, however, has been a problem for many tennis players. The top players are generally the ones who can control their thoughts and emotions on a consistent basis, which allows them to maintain a high level of excellence from day to day.

The remainder of the book will attempt to provide you with an in-depth approach to developing your mental skills. Understanding and taking control of your mental game will not only allow you to perform closer to your potential, but also make playing tennis an enjoyable and fun experience. The journey is not always an easy one, but the end result will provide you with the mental strength and psychological skills necessary to make your tennis experience not only more successful, but also more self-fulfilling.

CHAPTER 2

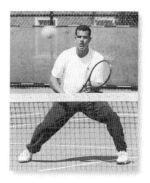

MENTAL STATES OF SUCCESSFUL TENNIS PLAYERS

Tennis players who are successful, tend to play up to their potential when it counts. But even the great players will sometimes fall prey to the ravages of the mind as they try hard to be at their best when it counts the most. So even the great Pete Sampras, who, to date, has won 13 Grand Slam titles, was less than his best in the 2000 and 2001 US Open finals against Marat Safin and Lleyton Hewitt (who both played great matches to win their first, and probably not last, Grand Slam title). When we play poorly (and this is usually attributed to something mental) this can initiate a vicious cycle of self-doubt, frustration, anger, self-criticism and disappointment. This cycle is not always easy to break (especially within a tennis match as opposed to across matches). This idea of not playing up to one's potential is explained in the following quote by two-time Grand Slam winner Rod Laver:

> *You can go out on the court some days and feel so sharp and so alert that the ball comes over the net looking as big as a soccer ball, and you think to yourself that there's no way I can make a mistake. Other days you can go out and play as if you're in a fog, unsure of everything. I can remember a match I played in Spain against Borg when my mind was miles away from the court and I had no real awareness of what I was doing except that I was getting beaten badly. The next day I played doubles and everything was back to normal. Can I explain the difference? I wish I could, but I can't. I can only say that tennis is a game you can never take for granted.*

> (Tarshis, 1977, p. 89)

Of course Rod Laver was "on" most of the time which helped make him one of the greatest champions of all time. But even the greatest players have days when their mind wanders and their play becomes erratic. Days can turn into weeks and months as Andre Agassi could probably attest to as he has certainly had an up and down career, based mainly on his mental outlook regarding tennis (of course becoming very physically fit is part of being mentally ready to play). Agassi has won all four different Grand Slams (played on clay, grass and hard court) and is the last player (male or female) to do so (presently the only current player). But he was ranked out of the top 100 and even played in Challenger matches in the mid to late 1990s to help bring his ranking back up, eventually reaching number 1 in the world. By his own admission, he lacked focus and motivation during these "down times" but all players know that when he is mentally and physically ready to play, he is one of the greatest players ever to play the game.

So how do we get ready to play every day when sometimes we are tired and sometimes we are playing a person who we believe is either a very easy or difficult opponent? Many tennis players often feel that they are on a performance roller coaster with a great performance one day followed by a sub-par performance the next. These players often do not know how they will perform on a given day and report that their mental and emotional states seem beyond their conscious control. Although we all, at times, feel out of control on the tennis court, there are many tennis players who never get a handle on their thoughts and emotions. This will usually result in increased frustration; the players eventually lose whatever interest and competitive drive they once possessed. Although this can occur at any age, junior players are particularly prone to this type of misfortune and we need to be sensitive to these situations for juniors.

Great Players are Consistent Players

The above analysis points toward consistency as one of the key characteristics of top performers. The distinguishing trademark of many of the top players past and present including Chris Evert, Mats Wilander, Martina Hingis, Ivan Lendl, Monica Seles, Steffi Graf, and Pete Sampras, was not so much their exceptional talent (although they all are very talented), but rather their exceptional ability to consistently play up to their capabilities whether week-to-week or in the Grand Slams. Almost anyone (with a fair amount of ability) can pull off a big upset on a given day or even get hot for an entire tournament like Goran Ivanisevic did for the 2001 Wimbledon Championships. But the bigger question is, can they maintain a high level of play over a period of time? You often hear about players scoring a big upset over a highly ranked opponent, only to fall in the next round or two to lesser opponents. An important part of the reason is that it is difficult to mentally stay focused and "at the top of your game" after spending so much mental and physical energy on beating a ranked opponent.

Along these lines, I have spoken to and worked with many players who erroneously evaluate their ability based on their best performance, such as beating the number 1 seed in a tournament or taking a top player to three sets before losing. More astute tennis players will realize, however, that they are only as good as their worst, not best day. In order to win a tournament, a player has to be able to withstand an off day and still find a way to win. The great champions do not let their games fall too much because they know that every match could result in an upset. A great victory is hollow if it's followed by a demoralizing defeat. Sometimes even top players struggle with consistency, especially after beating tough opponents. For example, in the 2001 US Open, Pete Sampras beat Patrick Rafter, Andre Agassi, and Marat Safin in successive rounds (all had previously won the US Open) and thus had little mental (and physical) energy left for his final with Lleyton Hewitt.

In an attempt to achieve consistency, two basic requirements are needed. First, a player needs good basic technique, stroke production, and movement. At the recreational level, many players are inconsistent simply because they have not sufficiently refined and practiced their strokes. Variability in one's mechanics, will lead to inconsistency in one's level of play. Even if you are mentally tough, inconsistencies will creep into your game if your stroke production and movement are inconsistent.

The second requirement for achieving consistency in your play, revolves around your mental and emotional skills. Sometimes you simply won't be able to play regularly due to work schedules, weather, or available court time, which may impact the consistency of your stroke production. But despite this, you should be able to control your mental state since it's not always directly related to on-court practice time. Thus, peaks and valleys in performance are many times related to psychological inconsistencies (especially when you are playing regularly). I think we all can relate to the fact that getting yourself in the proper psychological frame of mind and maintaining this state throughout a match is critical to success on the tennis court. But first, in order to get into the proper psychological state, a tennis player needs to know what this psychological state should be.

The Zone

I just started to feel so confident in my game. I felt that no matter how hard I hit the ball it was going to go in the court. I was no longer occupied with winning or losing, but rather I was just totally focused on the match.

Ivan Lendl after his victory over John McEnroe in the 1985 US Open
Dallas Morning News

Some people have a talent for serving and volleying. I have a talent for competing.
Jim Courier describing his mental toughness in matches

The above quotes from Lendl and Courier (both winners of multiple Grand Slams and formerly ranked number 1 in the world) describe how they felt in a particular match or in general regarding the mental side of their tennis games. In essence, Lendl describes a fleeting state, whereas Courier describes a more stable disposition, although both are important. This book could be filled with similar descriptions of other tennis players trying to recapture their thoughts and feelings relating to a particularly great performance or their sense of day-to-day mental toughness. It is interesting to note that when athletes in a variety of sports are asked to describe their top performances, they consistently use the same terminology and feeling states (Jackson & Csikszentimihalyi, 1999). In essence, there appears to be a unique psychological state that is associated with top performance. This mental state is distinctly different from the description of thoughts and feelings associated with poorer performance.

On a more scientific level, research evidence has been rapidly accumulating that links specific mental, physical, and emotional states of athletes during competition to the quality of their performance. The relationship between these special emotional and mental states and exceptional performance has been called peak experiences or flow. There has been a lot of terms used to describe this special state such as treeing, pumped, in the zone, in a groove, in the bubble, or on automatic pilot. Jim Loehr, noted sport psychologist working with top tennis players (and now top executives), uses the term Ideal Performance State to describe this constellation of special thoughts and feelings. I have chosen to use the term "in the zone" since this seems to be the most often used term to describe peak performance states by tennis players. This special mental state is not one in which players simply grit their teeth and "will" themselves to be mentally tough. So giving 110% effort (like many coaches request) will not bring about this elusive mental state. However, one of the basic premises of this book is that this state can be prepared for with specific mental training exercises. Along these lines, research with elite athletes has revealed that approximately 80% feel that this is a controllable state. This is not to say that a tennis player can easily get into this state; rather it says with proper training and technique, a tennis player can make it much more likely that he or she could reach such a mental state.

So if this state is not giving 100%, then what exactly is it? Playing in the zone usually means that the tennis player is so involved in the immediacy of the experience that he or she allows things to happen instead of trying to make them happen. As we shall see, it's like trying to relax. You can't really try to relax as much as relaxing by letting it happen or "letting go." Therefore, in this state, attention is directed externally to the immediate environment (e.g., the tennis ball or the movements of your opponent) to the virtual exclusion of one's own analytical thinking or other potential external distracters such as people watching the match. In essence, the body is reacting automatically and the player is just letting the body do what it is trained to do. There is no self-doubt, self-criticism, fear of failure, or other internal or external distracters, but rather a single-minded present focus.

A composite of the thoughts and feelings that tennis players report during outstanding or peak performance (i.e., in the zone) is presented on the following page:

I felt very relaxed, but yet I was energized and feeling strong. I enjoyed the tennis competition and was not afraid to lose. In fact I felt a sense of calmness and quiet inside, and my strokes just seemed to flow automatically. I really wasn't thinking about my shots and what I needed to do; it just seemed to happen naturally. My shots did not feel rushed, in fact the ball seemed to slow down and I felt as if I could do almost anything. I was totally into the match, but yet I was not consciously trying to concentrate. I was aware of everything but distracted by nothing. I knew no matter how hard I hit my shots they were going to go in. I felt confident and in total control.

Of course it is unusual for a tennis player to feel all of these things at one point in time, although it has been done. The key to what is generally called mental toughness is the ability to create and maintain the type of mental state described above. This special state can help bridge the gap between what you think you are capable of doing (what you can do) and what you actually do as a tennis player. In essence, the ability to "get in the zone" will allow you to perform consistently closer to your potential as a tennis player. You are always your toughest opponent and until you can win the battle of your mind, you will not consistently win the battle against your competition. The good news is that research has clearly shown that we all have the ability to control our thoughts and emotions which will help create the kind of internal climate that will allow us to get the most out of our physical skills and abilities. Much of this book will be dedicated to teaching you the skills necessary to achieve peak performance more regularly.

As noted earlier, these skills will need to be practiced like physical skills. But most competitive players spend a great amount of time practicing their physical skills (which is appropriate). What is not appropriate is the total lack of mental training on the part of many players, even though this does not require nearly the same amount of time as physical training. This special mental state is under your control; but you have to practice and develop the skills if you want to more consistently achieve high performance states. In essence, this book is not about 10 easy steps to improving your game and getting in the zone. But it is about increasing and sharpening the mental skills that get you ready to perform your best and reach your potential more often.

Thoughts and Feelings When "In the Zone"

There is now about 20-25 years of research systematically studying peak performance states of elite and recreational athletes (see Jackson & Csikszentimihalyi 1999 for a review). In depth interviews and paper and pencil inventories with athletes have come together to demonstrate that there are common mental and emotional states that athletes report when describing their top performances. I will now describe these states and then throughout the book, provide strategies and techniques to help tennis players achieve these special states.

Challenge-Skills Balance

One of the defining aspects of peak performance states is that there is a balance between a player's perceived skills and challenges. It's important to note that these skills and challenges are *perceived* by the player; in essence it's your subjective perception of skills and challenges that is most important. This means that it is not so much what the objective challenges or skills are in a situation that determines the quality of the experience, but what a person thinks of the available opportunities and of his or her capacity to act. Furthermore, it is not enough that challenges equal skills; both factors need to be extending the player to new levels. So when we play someone of equal ability where skills and challenges should be relatively matched (and this is how competition is purportedly set up) it is then more likely that a peak performance state will occur. However, we often find ourselves playing someone who is perceived to be somewhat better or worse than we are. But the sense of being in the zone most typically occurs when we are playing someone perceived to be better (as opposed to worse) than us (in essence, extending our skills to meet the challenge). How many times have you seen (or actually experienced) a player "playing up" when competing against an objectively better opponent. What often happens is that we try to bring our level of ability up to meet or match the difficult challenge. We can do this either by having more confidence in our own abilities (we'll speak more in depth about confidence later in the book), so that the challenge is matched, or possibly downplay the challenge somewhat ("my opponent is good but I can beat him if I play up to my potential").

When playing against a weaker opponent (the challenge is not equal to your ability), a good way to keep the challenge-skills balance is to set personal goals which are compared against your own standards of excellence. For example, you might try to achieve a first serve percentage of 65% compared to your average of 60%. Or you might want to achieve a 2-1 ratio of winners to unforced errors compared to a 1-1 ratio you normally have. We will discuss these performance goals in more detail in Chapter 4.

Action-Awareness Merging

This aspect of peak performance occurs when you feel at one with the movements you are making. Instead of the mind looking at the body from the outside as it were, the mind and body fuse into one. A tennis player describes what happens when he feels as though he has become one with his racquet:

> You don't really see yourself separate from the tennis racquet. It's like it's an extension of your arm. You feel like it's all just one piece working together. Strokes just happen in one smooth motion.

Action and awareness merge only when you become totally absorbed in what you are doing. This comes about when you feel that you have the skills to meet the challenges and when you focus all your attention at the task at hand. Athletes describe this total absorption in very positive terms such as, "everything feels very smooth and fluid," or "I'm in the groove." A tennis player described it as "I'm totally absorbed in my stroke." Tennis players and other athletes report that actions seem effortless and spontaneous. Even though a player might be making a superhuman effort, at the moment it feels entirely natural. As a professional tennis player said, "Things just happen automatically. I just am hitting the ball, but not really thinking about it."

When describing this action-awareness merging, athletes note the sensation of floating, and of things feeling easy. A sense of ease of movement is often mentioned as the athlete experiences changed perceptions of effort and their physical body in space. For example, tennis can oftentimes be an arduous and even painful experience as one gets tired and sore from a long grueling match. But tennis players (and other athletes) have been able to overcome this sense of pain, fatigue, and aching muscles, and enter an effortless rhythm that transforms their agony into ecstasy. This is part of being "in the zone." Many top athletes such as Michael Jordan, Wayne Gretsky, and Tiger Woods, as well top tennis players such as Monica Seles, Andre Agassi, and Venus Williams, all talk about the playing field or court as being the one place of refuge from day-to-day concerns and demands, where they can become totally absorbed in the competition and forget about everything else. Although I will discuss strategies later, some potential ways of helping to become totally absorbed in the activity include: (a) forgetting yourself and your ego, in essence a loss of self-consciousness; (b) focus on the process, not the outcome; and (c) accept, don't evaluate the environment.

Feelings of Confidence

Many researchers have investigated the differences between successful and less successful athletes. Although several differences emerge, one of the key characteristics of elite performers is their strong belief in themselves, despite what might be seen as a poor performance. For tennis players, this belief would transcend any particular point, game, set or match. In essence, your confidence is not going to be shaken just because you play poorly one day or get beat easily in a given match. Some athletes refer to this unwavering confidence in terms of "feelings of control." In a sense, they feel that they can do no-wrong which is consistent with descriptions of tennis players who describe themselves feeling "unbeatable," "like I can do anything." More than actually being in control, it is the feeling of being in control, and that you have the skills to perform the task successfully. This sense of control helps build your confidence because you know that you can get the job done.

Every tennis player is gong to have "off" days where things just don't seem to go right and you're out of your normal rhythm. However, the great champions do not let these setbacks undermine their genuine belief that they can and will be successful. This can even happen within a match or a set where a player could start off poorly but turn things around because he kept his confidence in his abilities to make shots and win the match. The following quote will illustrate the central role that confidence plays in one's tennis game.

When you're not confident it affects nearly everything you do on the court; the way you move, the way you hit the ball, the way you think. You let winning opportunities go by, you tighten up on easy points; it's the catalyst to your entire game. When it goes your game goes.

(Tarshis, 1977, p. 91)

Stan Smith, former number 1 ranked tennis player in the world

Confidence affects the way you strike the ball and if you go for your shots or "play it safe." As one touring professional tennis player has said "the difference between feeling confident and not feeling confident is that you never hesitate to go for shots when you're confident, but you tend to be tentative and just try to keep the ball in play when you're not feeling confident." Confidence is typically brought into the picture whenever tennis players talk about playing well or playing poorly. For example, you invariably hear comments such as, "I just didn't have confidence in my strokes today" or, conversely, " I felt really confident out there, like everything I hit was going in the court." Since confidence is such a critical factor to a tennis player's success, we will discuss it in greater depth in a later chapter.

Focused Concentration

When tennis players describe their top or peak performances, they invariably talk about being totally focused on the match. They are totally focused on the present and do not think about the past or future. In addition, they do not pay attention to, or sometimes are not even aware of, distractions in the immediate environment. For example, a player may be totally unaware of the behavior of the crowd since she is so focused in on their opponent and the ball. Tennis is a game that can go on for several hours and possibly one lapse in concentration (such as on a break point) could mean the difference between winning and losing. This fine line and importance of focused concentration over time is highlighted in the following quote by the great champion, Bjorn Borg.

Very often in a tennis match you can point to just one point or game where for a couple of shots you lost concentration and didn't do the right thing, and the difference in the match will be right there.

(Tarshis, 1977, p. 21)

It is interesting to note that many tennis players, when describing their best performances, report that they are not really trying to concentrate; rather, concentration seems to happen naturally. In essence, it's difficult to force concentration (and we'll see the same phenomenon for relaxation). However, it is not likely that focused concentration will simply happen if you do not practice concentration skills. In fact this is one of the key foundation points of this book—that mental skills need to be practiced and developed just like physical skills. The notion of practicing concentration skills is highlighted by the following quote by Chris Evert, who was noted for her extraordinary concentration skills.

Basically, what my dad and I used to do in my practice sessions was to keep hitting as many balls as we could without a miss. With me, concentration developed so naturally that I rarely had to force myself to do it. It was just part of my game.

(Tarshis, 1977, p. 32)

It is difficult to keep concentration focused throughout a tennis match. The longer each point goes and the longer a match goes, the more important concentration becomes. Add on things such as wind, noise, sun, line calls, and opponent's antics, and it becomes obvious that a player without good concentration skills is doomed to failure. For this reason, proper attentional focus is discussed in more detail later in the book.

Clear Goals

Another aspect of this special performance state is that athletes have clear goals. Goals help direct action and focus and it is important for tennis players to know where they are headed both in the short term and long term. To enter the zone, tennis players need to set goals clearly in advance, so that they know exactly what to do. When athletes describe optimal sport experiences, two themes related to goals stand out. The first is a clear blueprint of what one is supposed to do illustrated by the following statement: " I knew exactly what I needed to do to win the tennis match and beat my opponent." Brad Gilbert, in his book, *Winning Ugly*, oftentimes notes that in order for him to compete against and possibly beat players with more physical ability, he had to have a specific plan and know what strokes to hit and what areas to attack. In essence, when he got out on the court he knew exactly what he needed to do to be successful.

Clear goals are also important, since psychological well-being requires full involvement of the entire person; without clear demands on attention, the mind begins to turn towards different areas of one's life (such as what you will be doing later, or what a friend said to you). As a result, productivity decreases, as energy is not directed in specific and purposeful ways on the tennis court. So, for example, if a player is practicing without a specific goal, then she tends to hit the ball back over the net to her partner without really working on a particular stroke or strategy. All too often, practice becomes monotonous and players go through the motions of playing but really don't accomplish anything. So whether it's practice or matches, clear goals help focus a player on what needs to be done and then on doing it. We'll speak about how to set effective goals in Chapter 4.

Loss of Self-Consciousness

Many tennis players are concerned about what others think of them (especially if they lose or play poorly). They don't want to disappoint friends, coaches, and parents or let themselves down. Unfortunately, thoughts of letting people down, losing, and making mistakes often occupy players' minds before, during, and after matches. However, when describing peak performances, tennis players' concern for the self disappears, as do worries or negative thoughts. There is simply no attention left over to worry about things that in everyday life we usually spend so much time dwelling on. In essence, when a tennis player is in the zone, he or she is freed from self-concern and self-doubt. There is no fear; rather, the player is calm and quiet inside. Many players play not to lose instead of playing to win (especially when they are ahead or are beating a more highly ranked opponent) and this usually results in tentative play and holding back on their shots. Tennis great, Chris Evert never really had this "play not to lose" thinking in her mental approach to tennis as illustrated by the following quote.

> *A lot of it really had to do with the way I was raised. My father was very careful to react pretty much the same way whether I won or lost. When he was critical, it was never because of the outcome of the match, but because of certain things I may not have done right. But he was never harsh. I never went into a match afraid of how he would react if I lost.*
>
> *(Tarshis, 1977, p. 76)*

This loss of self-consciousness is related to feeling loose and relaxed on the tennis court. Research has indicated that tennis players usually perform at their best when they are physically relaxed with a minimum of muscle tension. Tight muscles cause a player to lose the fluidity and timing in their strokes and they start to "push" the ball and become tentative the more they tighten up. Relaxed muscles allow you to hit topspin and come over the ball in order to impart the proper spin to help keep the ball in play. Tight muscles cause you to lose the spin and hit the ball long. Besides messing up coordination, consistent muscle tension is fatiguing, especially in long matches. As the great Arthur Ashe once pointed out:

> *The one thing I've learned about tension on the court that's helped me is something I got from Pancho Gonzalez. He told me once that if you can somehow learn to relax between points, the tension won't build up in a match the way it does if you try to concentrate every second. Physical fatigue can make you mentally tired and whatever you do to minimize the tension will make choking less likely.*
>
> *(Tarshis, 1977, p. 87)*

Therefore, the notion of being able to relax will be discussed in Chapter 5. A key here is to lose your self-consciousness (not your consciousness) and not be concerned about how others might evaluate how you look or how you play. If you can do this, then your strokes will become more automatic with a minimum of thinking about how to hit the ball. As Tim Gallwey (1974) has noted in his classic, *Inner Game of Tennis*, a player in the zone knows where he wants the ball to go, but he doesn't have to try hard to get it there. When, after playing really well, players sometimes say they were "unconscious out there." But what they are really saying is that their minds were so concentrated and focused that they put their bodies on automatic pilot with no interference from thoughts and emotions. One of the major goals of this book is to help each of you reach this state of mind more often.

Intrinsic Motivation (Enjoyment)

One of the basic qualities of peak performance is that it typically occurs when one is intrinsically motivated to play and derives a great deal of enjoyment from competing. In essence, a player is competing against another player simply because they are having fun (even though they might be receiving extrinsic rewards such as money and publicity). This sense of playing for the love of the game was noted about Pete Sampras after he had already broken the record with his 13th Grand Slam title. Some people were feeling that he was not sufficiently motivated to win any more Grand Slams especially in light of his marriage, achievement of the Grand Slam record, and 6 years as the number 1 ranked player in the world. But here is where the love of the game might be paramount. As former number 1 player Stan Smith said of Sampras:

> If he can continue to really have a love for the game, which he seems to do, then the only thing that could affect him are his other activities.

Rod Laver says something similar about Sampras:

> If he keeps his love for the game he'll keep winning. It's got to be a joy to go out there and play.

Finally, Pete Sampras himself sounds a similar note about his motivation:

> You have to do what makes you happy. If I feel like I am not having fun out there on the court, it is time to do something else.

This idea of having fun is echoed by Pete Sampras' long time rival Andre Agassi:

> Sometimes I find myself getting a little too serious. When I'm having fun, it breaks the tension and I play much better.

On the flip side, many tennis players burn out (especially young players) because they have lost the fun and enthusiasm for the game. This fact has been highlighted by recent research by Gould and his colleagues (1997) who studied burnout in youth tennis players and found that losing the enjoyment and fun of playing was a prime reason for leaving the game. This might have been due to excessive time on the court, training regimens, travel schedules, boring practices, pressured environments, negative feedback from parents and coaches, or some combination of the above. But no matter what the reason, the final result was that they lost their love for tennis. To be good at tennis requires a lot of hard work, dedication, and practice and thus the successful tennis player must be motivated to train hard and practice. Although there have been some highly visible top young tennis players who have said they have suffered from burnout, there is a large number of competitive junior players who simply lose their love of the game by the time they reach college age. Since tennis can be a lifetime sport, it is extremely unfortunate that relatively young players are giving up the game and becoming burned out. This lack of fun, eventually leading to burnout, is captured in the following quote by a young tennis player.

> *I used to look forward to getting up in the morning so I could play tennis. I couldn't wait to get on the tennis court because it was so much fun and I really enjoyed it. But as time passed by it became more and more difficult for me to get motivated to play whether in practice or in a match. I'm not sure if it was the pressure of winning, the boredom of practice, the same players in the same tournaments, or just my feeling that there are other things in life beside hitting a tennis ball over a net. Whatever the reason, I just lost my spark and enthusiasm and tennis has become a drag—more like work than play.*

So what makes tennis fun for you? On a piece of paper, list the factors that make tennis fun for you as well as the things that take away the fun and contribute to burning out from tennis. Throughout the book, we will be discussing how to make tennis a more enjoyable experience for all players.

Assessing Mental Skills

Thus far, this chapter has emphasized that consistent, high-level play will most often be accomplished if you can first consistently create the proper internal mental state or as we say, get "in the zone." When the right internal state takes form, playing well seems to occur naturally and spontaneously. We have noted that the most recent research indicates that these peak performance states include the following:

- Balance of Skill and Challenges
- Merging of Action and Awareness
- High Levels of Confidence
- Focused Concentration
- Clear Goals
- Loss of Self-Consciousness
- Enjoyment-Motivation

One of the most important aims of this book is to help players get into this special state more consistently. Along these lines, I will now provide an assessment tool to help you better understand your strengths and weaknesses, especially from a mental standpoint.

Performance Profiling

A fairly recent technique termed *performance profiling* has been developed (Butler & Hardy, 1992) to both identify important mental skills training objectives and help maximize the motivation of athletes to implement and adhere to a mental skills training program. To use this technique, tennis players would first be asked to identify the characteristics or qualities (specifically mental) of elite tennis players. The tennis player would list all of the qualities on a piece of paper (this also could be done with teams asking all players to list qualities of top tennis players through brainstorming in small groups). In essence, this could be done by you, as an individual player, or by your coach. In a team situation, after the players stopped writing, coaches might assist players in identifying other characteristics by mentioning qualities noted by other top tennis players. A player would then rate herself (on a 1-10 scale representing the degree to which the player feels she has the mental skills of top tennis players) on all the qualities that she identified and her responses would be translated into a "Performance Profile" (see Figure 2.1), providing a visual representation of the player's strengths and potential areas of improvement. This approach is particularly effective since the player is generating the key mental concepts and does a self-rating as to which areas need improvement. For example, on the sample profile provided, the player feels that she is doing well (although, of course, she could always do better) in the areas of visualization, mental preparation and communication, but could use a good deal of improvement in managing anxiety, confidence, concentration, and self-talk. So if you were this player, you might pay particular attention to these areas and chapters as you read through the book. In addition, on a separate piece of paper, you might list some of the things you could do to improve these weaker areas. These could then be compared with some of the techniques and strategies presented later in this book. Take some time to complete this assessment to determine where you stand in relation to the pros regarding these critical skills.

Becoming Mentally Tough

The primary goal of the ensuing chapters is to help you develop and learn your mental skills to the point where you can control your mental and emotional states instead of them being in control of you. Being a mentally tough tennis player translates into the ability to create and maintain the proper psychological state regardless of the situation or circumstances. But what are the actual qualities of mentally tough tennis players? In a recent study (Jones, Hanton, & Connauughton, 2002) 10 international level tennis players were extensively interviewed to help define what mentally tough really is (at least in their eyes). The top attributes in ranked order were as follows:

• Having an unshakable self-belief in your ability to achieve your competition goals.
• Bouncing back from performance setbacks as a result of increased determination.

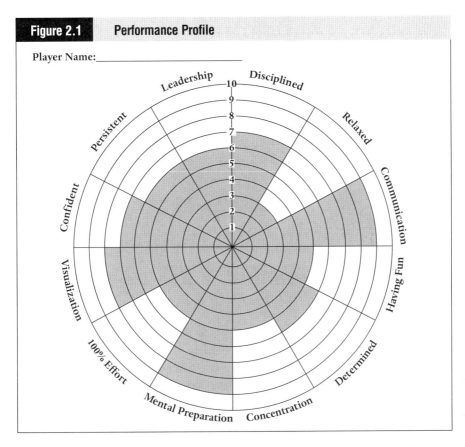

Figure 2.1   Performance Profile

Player Name:_____

- Having an unshakable self-belief that you possess unique qualities and abilities that make you better than your opponent.
- Remaining fully focused on the task at hand in the face of competition-specific distractions.
- Having a strong desire and internalized motives to succeed.
- Regaining psychological control following unexpected, uncontrollable events.

Although stated in somewhat different terms, these attributes are generally similar to the ones described earlier in this chapter regarding optimal psychological states for peak performance. As you probably realize, these states are easier to maintain when things are going your way on the court. The real test is when things get tough, the pressure gets high, you're behind, and everything seems to be going wrong. If you can stay confident, focused, relaxed and motivated under these difficult circumstances, then you are well on the way to winning the mental game. It won't always be easy, but when you get there, it will have been one of the most satisfying journeys of your life.

CHAPTER 3

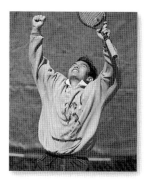

ASSESSING AND IMPROVING COMMITMENT

Now that you know some of the mental states that are consistently associated with peak performance and being "in the zone" the next step is to make sure that you are committed to action. Being committed means different things to different people. The following quote by a ranked junior tennis player sums up one way to view commitment.

> *I would get up every morning ready to play tennis. I would play several hours every day, whether I could find someone to play with, just hit against the wall, practice serving, or go against a ball machine. In practice I would always go the extra yard and run the sprints harder, practice with focused concentration and intensity, or stay after practice for extra work. I was committed to getting better and was willing to make the sacrifices necessary to get to the next level.*

Another way to view commitment comes from Thomas Edison and his attempt to invent the filament for a light bulb. He documented more than 10,000 different attempts until he invented a filament that would burn for a reasonable length of time. He was later asked, *"How did it feel to fail 10,000 times in your experiments?"* He replied, *"I didn't fail 10,000 times. I just found out 10,000 ways that didn't work."*

These quotes capture many of the elements of commitment including intensity, effort, perspective and persistence. Some of the terms associated with commitment include drive, desire, heart, attitude, persistence, intensity, hustle and sacrifice. But in a simpler sense, commitment is basically striving toward a goal with great intensity (we will discuss goals in

Chapter 4). Players with higher levels of commitment, usually continue to strive to reach their goals despite obstacles placed in their way. In essence, committed players tolerate pain and frustration more, practice more, play with more intensity, and persist in the face of failure. Martina Navratilova aptly sums up being committed with the following quote.

> *With motivation you can be involved or committed. Just like with ham and eggs; the chicken was involved, but the pig was committed. You have to be like the pig.*

Assessing Commitment

One way of evaluating your own level of commitment is to complete the self-help test provided in Table 3.1. Although the scores are merely suggestive (you should also consider your actual behaviors), there are some general guidelines regarding your score. For example, scores in the 40s or higher suggest a very high level of commitment. Some people have argued that such high levels of commitment represent an imbalance in someone's personality or some kind of fanaticism. This is a tough question as some tennis players appear extremely committed and sometimes sacrifice their personal lives, their finances, and even their health in pursuit of tennis success. You will notice that most top professional tennis players remain single throughout their prime years due, at least in part, to the single mindedness and total commitment it takes to make it make it to the top and stay there.

Andre Agassi is just one case in point. Agassi married Brooke Shields and his commitment to tennis obviously fell, as did his ranking. When he split up with Brooke Shields and recommitted himself to tennis, he again became one of the top players in the world. He even played in some Challenger events to help build his confidence and commitment. This is not to argue that it is better to be totally focused on your tennis and to leave your personal life behind. Rather, decisions have to be made regarding balancing your commitment to tennis against other important aspects of your life (we will talk about making decisions later in the chapter). Some people prefer a nice balance between their personal and tennis lives and even say that the social support they receive from their spouse is critical to help keep up that level of commitment. Other people prefer to be totally focused on tennis (although that, at times, can lead to burnout—this will be discussed later in the book). They feel they need a single-mindedness about improving and working on their games and to at least put off forming significant relationships until later in their tennis careers (perhaps when they have achieved, or at least approached, their tennis goals). Only you can make that kind of decision regarding focusing on tennis versus developing enduring personal relationships. but you should be aware of the potential consequences of your commitment (or lack of commitment).

Table 3.1	Tennis Commitment Self-Help Test

Read each of the items below carefully. For each item, insert a number from 1 to 5 next to the item by deciding which of the following alternatives most accurately describes your current feelings about that item.

5 = Extremely characteristic of me
4 = Somewhat characteristic of me
3 = Neither characteristic nor uncharacteristic of me
2 = Somewhat uncharacteristic of me
1 = Extremely uncharacteristic of me

Commitment

_____1. I am very committed to tennis.

_____2. I am good at keeping my promise to practice tennis.

_____3. Even when I find tennis difficult to do, I try especially hard to stick with it.

_____4. I will persist at tennis despite pain, discomfort, or inconvenience.

_____5. I am determined to reach my goals in tennis.

_____6. Regarding tennis, I will not let myself down.

_____7. I am very eager to develop the kind of self-discipline I need to participate in tennis to the best of my ability.

_____8. Sometimes I push myself harder than I should when practicing or competing in tennis.

_____9. I have a lot of willpower to participate and master tennis.

_____10. I will persist at practicing and competing in tennis despite occasional failures.

_____Commitment Total

Factors That Increase Initial Commitment

You might be one of those people who are not sure whether you should really commit yourself to tennis or not. Later in the chapter we will take a look at a decision balance sheet technique that might help you make this decision. But for now, let's examine some of the factors that encourage people to make commitments (see Kirschenbaum,1997 for a more detailed discussion of commitment).

Actual Change not Required Until the Future

Most people will feel a stronger desire to commit, if they view that the changes required wouldn't go into effect until sometime in the future. For example, I was working with a tennis player who needed to improve her commitment if she was going to get to the next level. But this would require an increased amount of time practicing and working on specific physical and mental skills. Since the main tennis season for her was over (which meant the spring and summer) we decided to start her new regimen in two months. She knew that she was kind of burned out on tennis now, but was willing to renew her commitment to increased time on and off the court in a couple of months. Although it may seem like stalling, players generally will commit to something in the near future rather than put something into action right now.

History of Making Promises a Reality

You have all heard the term "talk is cheap." Some people talk a good game while others act on their promises. People with a history of following through on their commitments are more likely to follow-through on new commitments. In essence, the best predictor of future behavior is past behavior. You should take pride in making good on your promises and this also provides a sense of self-satisfaction. So make tennis one of your commitments for the future, but don't make your promises larger than you can realistically achieve.

Recent "Peak Performance" Experiences

Remember from Chapter 2 that athletes are, at least in part, in control of their peak performances. If you have recently had a peak performance in tennis, you are more likely to stay committed to the sport. For example, if you really played at the top of your game in recent weeks, it provides added motivation for you to stay committed to your tennis over time. The positive feeling states that typically accompany peak performances, help tennis players stay motivated and committed, since it is just flat out enjoyable to feel this way after a top performance. And remember, you can put yourself in the right frame of mind to experience these positive emotions by controlling your thoughts and feelings prior to performance (many of the subsequent chapters in the book will help you learn this type of control).

Mastering Difficult Skills

One of the things that gets athletes committed and keeps them committed is the possibility of mastering (or at least successfully completing on occasion) very difficult skills. One of the great thrills in sports is being able to master a very difficult shot or play or being able to compete with (and possibly beat) a very talented opponent. The joy of competing and meeting special challenges certainly can enhance commitment. For example, many people were amazed that Michael Jordan would attempt a comeback even though he left the game making a basket to win a championship and is arguably the greatest player ever to play basketball. So what else was there to prove? But it wasn't about proving things to others or possibly spoiling a reputation that could only be considered legendary. What it was about was meeting a new challenge—could he still be great at age 38? (the answer is a resounding YES—at the time of the release of this book, he was leading the long downtrodden

Washington Wizards back to respectability with his inspired play). This emphasizes not only the love of the sport, but also a commitment to excellence and meeting new challenges.

Taking the Michael Jordan example and the principle of meeting challenges in the tennis world, it would appear that your commitment could be enhanced by emphasizing the potential challenges ahead, as well as the feelings of satisfaction of mastering certain skills. For example, your practices could be set up in such a way as to increase commitment and motivation by providing challenging activities (this is similar to the skill-challenge balance discussed in Chapter 2 regarding peak performance states). In addition, for many tennis players, commitment is increased, simply by striving to master difficult skills. And you can make skills as difficult as you want simply by changing your goals (which we'll discuss in the next chapter). For example, a first serve becomes more difficult if you draw a line halfway between the net and service line and try to hit the ball between the line and service line (getting depth on your serve). Similarly, a simple forehand becomes more difficult to master if you have a goal of hitting 10 in a row down the line, within 3 feet of the sideline and past the service line. Of course the possibilities are endless, but make sure your challenges are in relation to your current skill level.

Being Around Others Who Make Commitments to Change

It is important to surround yourself with people who share a commitment to tennis. When you are around others who are working hard and striving toward excellence, it makes things just that much easier for you to commit. For example, you might not be in the mood to practice but you're scheduled to hit with a good friend of yours who has been working hard on his game and is committed to improving his tennis. So you go out there (even though you might not have if it weren't for your friend) and the motivation and effort of your friend rubs off on you and you start practicing hard, putting forth lots of effort and energy. In addition, your friend is supportive of your efforts to improve and encourages you to stay committed, since there will be positive results and outcomes down the road.

Making a Commitment Leads to Immediate Benefits

Although sometimes making a commitment to improve your game, win a club championship, practice 3 times a week, or improve your sectional ranking can be difficult, it usually is met with a lot of immediate positive benefits. For example, declaring your commitment to significant others such as parents, coaches, teammates, or friends, will typically produce shows of encouragement and support of your decision. People generally appreciate and value when one is committed to a particular course of action and will provide positive feedback or get excited about this commitment.

I remember working with a young tennis player who was talented (ranked highly in the juniors), but yet floundering due to lack of motivation and commitment. After a couple of sessions, she agreed to commit to play regularly again (3-4 times per week) and to give full effort both mentally and physically to her time on the court. When she was off the court, we agreed that she should focus on her other activities. We devised a training plan that would challenge her and maximize her motivation by combining some basic drilling with some innovative drills and activities that she saw as fun, but yet challenging. Once she made this commitment, both her coach and her parents got really excited to see her back on the court and working hard. Their excitement spilled over outside of tennis, and this in turn increased the player's commitment to practice hard and improve her game. In fact, she wound up getting a college scholarship and had a very successful (and fun) four years of varsity tennis.

Improving Commitment

I have briefly discussed six factors that have consistently been related to improving commitment. In addition, you have had the opportunity to take a brief inventory to give you a sense of where you fall regarding your sense of commitment to tennis. However, research also clearly supports the use of a couple of other techniques and strategies that have demonstrated their usefulness in enhancing commitment.

Decision Balance Sheet

One way that people make commitments is to simply weigh the potential positive outcomes for making the change versus the negative outcomes of not making the change. One thing you could do is simply list the positive and negative factors regarding increasing your commitment to tennis (that's if you think you are not committed enough right now and possibly need to be more committed). Or you could be a little more specific and list the pros and cons of becoming committed to a specific goal in tennis such as improving your first serve (maybe it's percentage, speed, placement, or all of the above).

To make the decision, of improving the percentage, placement, and speed of your first serve (we'll talk next chapter about how to state your goals), we will use a strategy known as a *Decision Balance Sheet*, which was developed more than 25 years ago but has been used to help enhance commitment of both exercise and sport behaviors. In our decision, we would consider practicing the serve for an extra half hour after the normal practice is concluded. Table 3.2 presents a sample Decision Balance Sheet for improving your first serve. Notice that you are focusing on three things: (a) benefits/drawbacks to yourself; (b) self-approval/disapproval; and (c) social approval/disapproval. In essence, you are considering not only yourself, but also others.

After putting down your reasons in the different categories, you should carefully review your positive and negative outcomes. But this is not just a matter of adding up the positives versus the negatives, with more responses leading to your decision. For example, in the illustration provided, there are obviously more positive than negative outcomes both to yourself and others, regarding making a commitment to improving your first serve. But

Table 3.2	Decision Balance Sheet for Improving Your First Serve	

Gains to Self
Improve my tennis serve
Feel good about my game
Win more matches
Enjoy practice more
I'll become a better player

Losses to Self
Increased time spent practicing the serve
Increased money taking lessons
Repetition of serve –maybe boring
Time away from friends

Self Approval
I'll feel proud if I succeed
I'll understand my game a bit more
I'll learn about the serving process
I feel excited about the challenge
I'd feel a sense of accomplishment

Self Disapproval
Frustration if I fail
Increased pressure to improve
Worrying about the serve

Social Approval
My coach will be proud
My teammates will admire me
My parents will admire my dedication

Social Disapproval
Teammates will kid me if I fail
Friends will think I'm obsessive

Very Important Items From Your Decision Balance Sheet

Positive Items (to self and others)	Negative Items (to self and others)
_____	_____
_____	_____
_____	_____

this should not automatically lead you to the conclusion to make the commitment and decision to practice your first serve as described earlier. Specifically, you also have to consider how important each item is to you. So you might rate each of the items that you listed from "1" (unimportant) to "2" (important) to "3" (very important). This will further help you decide on the best course of action.

For instance, in the examples provided, if you put down that improving your tennis game, winning more matches, and becoming a better player, were all very important to you, while nothing on the negative side was very important to you, then the decision to commit to work on your serve, would seem to be a reasonable one, based on the decision balance sheet. But if a couple of the negatives were also very important, then the decision would be more difficult. But the big advantage is that you can look in very objective terms regarding the outcomes that the decision to commit to a particular behavior have on you and others, and then go and make an informed decision about pursuing this commitment.

Challenging Excuse Making

People tend to rationalize their decisions, especially when these decisions go against common sense or accumulated evidence. For example, have you ever discussed a cigarette habit with a smoker? You may have heard him or her say such things as, "I know someone who smoked two packs a day and is still alive at 80, while someone I know who ran almost every day and stayed in great shape died at age 50." Or, "What's the big deal about smoking. I could get run over by a bus crossing the street—life is a risk."

It's amazing that providing justification for one's behavior is just as typical of athletes as non-athletes. Many athletes make excuses regarding why they are out of shape, why they haven't practiced regularly, or why they aren't improving. They sometimes blame the coach, sometimes it's teammates, and sometimes it's just the environment that they can't control (e.g., too hot, too cold, too windy). It's easy to put off to tomorrow what you could have done today. The problem is that this can easily become a habit. Then you find yourself routinely putting off things and you always have a convenient excuse for not doing something now.

Of course, tennis players are not immune to making excuses. In my years of playing and coaching tennis, as well as consulting with many tennis players, I have found a number of typical reasons that players give for not practicing hard, not physically training hard (fitness), not working on a particular stroke(s) or avoiding practice completely. In Table 3.3 I have listed the 10 top excuses that tennis players make for not working hard or putting in the required effort to be successful. So please take the self-help test provided in Table 3.3 following the instructions. If you total 30 or more, you tend to use excuses quite frequently in avoiding workouts or not trying hard in practices. This excuse making would typically be seen in actual behavioral differences, with tennis players scoring lower on this scale, more likely to put forth consistent effort during practices and practice hard both on and off the court to improve their tennis games. So where do you stand in regards to excuse-making?

In working with young tennis players, I try to get them to counter or dispute these excuses. If you can dispute your excuses, then it becomes easier to stay committed to follow a course of action. So a good exercise is to look at the excuses that are particularly relevant to you and develop disputing responses for each of these excuses. This is a little like changing negative to positive self-talk, which we will discuss in Chapter 9. In Table 3.4, I provide examples of some disputing responses to common excuses and then let you develop responses specific to you for the other excuses. If you can develop some specific responses to your excuse-making (if you are an excuse-maker), then research has revealed that you can boost your chances of re-igniting your commitment to tennis.

Table 3.3	Excuses for Not Training and Practicing for Tennis

The following is a list of statements that tennis players often give when they consider working out and training to improve their tennis games. Please read each statement carefully. Then, next to each statement, indicate how frequently you made this statement during the past month using the following scale:

1 = Not at all
2 = Sometimes
3 = Moderately often
4 = Often
5 = All the time

Frequency	Reason
_____	I'm too tired.
	I'm too busy.
	I have more important things to do.
_____	I'll do it tomorrow.
_____	I really don't need to play or workout.
_____	I just want to take the day off.
_____	It's no big deal if I miss one day.
_____	I'm just not motivated today.
_____	I just don't feel like playing.
_____	I need to just recuperate.

Becoming Committed (Or Becoming More Committed)

After reading this chapter and completing the exercises, you should have a pretty good idea of your commitment to tennis as well as specific strategies for enhancing commitment. So start by taking the commitment scale in Table 3.1 to get a read on your level of commitment. Then understand the factors related to becoming more committed. To be sure of your commitment to specific goals in tennis, go through the Decision-Balance Sheet in Table 3.2. Finally, Tables 3.3 and 3.4 allow you to understand the typical excuses that are made to not train and play tennis and how to dispute some of these excuses. You now should be re-energized and ready to set some goals in your tennis life.

Table 3.4 **Typical Tennis Excuses and Some Disputing Responses**

Tennis Excuses	Disputing Responses
I'm too tired.	Playing tennis will energize me. I am unwilling to give in to a temporary feeling of tiredness.
I have more important things to do.	Making time for my tennis is as important as anything else. Tennis helps me in lots of ways both on and off the court—especially to be disciplined.
I'm too busy.	Tennis does take time but I'm investing in myself. Tennis keeps me fit and healthy and feeling good.
I'll do it tomorrow.	I made time in my day to do it today. It may not happen tomorrow. Do it now—I'll feel better for it.
I really don't need to play today.	_____
I just want to take the day off.	_____
It's no big deal if I miss one day.	_____
I'm just not motivated today.	_____
I just don't feel like playing.	_____
I need to just recuperate.	_____

CHAPTER 4

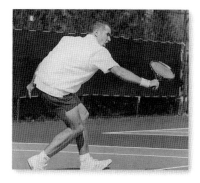

MOTIVATION THROUGH EFFECTIVE GOAL-SETTING

In Chapter 3 we discussed the importance of being committed and motivated for long term development and improvement as a tennis player, and you should have found out something about your commitment and motivation through the self-help tests provided. But now we need to try to enhance that motivation to improve, compete, and practice. One tried and true way to keep motivation high and focus one's attention on the task at hand is through the use of goal-setting. Simply knowing what you want (e.g., winning your club championship) is not enough; you need to have specific plans and goals in order to reach your desired outcomes. The following quote by a collegiate tennis player captures the important role that goals can have on a tennis player's motivation.

Motivation depends in a very large part on goal setting. The coach must have goals. The team must have goals. Each individual tennis player must have goals, real, vivid, living goals... Goals keep everyone on target. Goals commit me to the work, time, pain and whatever else is part of the price of achieving success.

Although the mental skills that will be presented in subsequent chapters are all important for ultimately achieving your best on the tennis court, without proper motivation, you will only go so far. Goals can play a critical role in sustaining motivation and providing you with a sense of direction and purpose as well as stimulating you to meet challenges. As Keith Bell (1983) aptly noted in his book entitled *Championship Thinking*, "Floundering in the world of sports without setting goals is like shooting without aiming. You might enjoy the blast and kick of the gun, but you probably won't bag the bird."

The focus of this chapter is to get you more familiar with the principles of effective goal setting. First, I will provide a definition of goal setting (including different types of goals) as well as identifying why goals work. Second, I will discuss some of the key principles for effective goal setting. Third, I will present a goal-setting system for both coaches and players to implement.

Definition and Types of Goals

In the scientific literature, a goal is typically defined as an objective, a standard, an aim, or a level of performance or proficiency. Some people focus on more objective goals such as improving your first serve percentage from 50% to 60%, or improving your winners to unforced error percentage from 50% (e.g. 10 winners to 20 unforced errors) to 75% (15 winners to 20 unforced errors). These objective goals can be very specific such as hitting 10 consecutive ground strokes past the service line but in the court, or more general such as winning the club championship. Although more difficult, other people focus on subjective goals, such as having more fun or improving concentration (these are harder to measure but are just as important as objective goals). The definition of a goal also implies that these performance (or mental) standards will be accomplished within some specified period of time such as a week or a month. Our focus will be more on objective goals (or at least trying to quantify goals in an objective manner so we know if we are approaching or have reached our goal). We will now review the three major types of goals including outcome, performance and process goals.

Outcome Goals

Outcome goals typically focus on the outcome of a competitive event such as winning a match, winning a specific tournament, being ranked number 4 in your region, or achieving a 12-6 record for a season as a coach. Thus, achieving these goals depends not only on your ability and efforts, but also on the ability and play of your opponents. In essence, you are not really in control of achieving outcome goals since it depends, at least in part, on the performance of others. For example, you might play the best match of your life and still lose a tough match 5-7, 7-6, 5-7, since your opponent also was playing "in the zone." Thus, you might not have achieved your goal of winning the match. Conversely, you might have not played up to your potential but played a weaker opponent who also was off his game, and you squeaked out a victory 6-4, 6-7, 7-5. Should you feel happy with your performance just because you won the match and reached your goal?

Sport psychologists (supported by research) generally do not favor a sole focus on outcome goals (and unfortunately many tennis players–as well as other athletes "put all their eggs in the outcome basket") since they are not under one's control. In addition, they can lead to frustration, disappointment, increased anxiety, lack of trying, and a focus on irrelevant, distracting thoughts, such as worrying too much about the outcome of the match, instead of what you need to do to play well and win points. But our society sees success in sports as a highly valued goal, and success to most athletes and coaches (as well as parents) simply means winning. So as tennis players mature and get better, they focus on competitive outcomes and how well they are doing in relation to others. Therefore, winning trophies, being highly ranked in the juniors, and winning matches becomes more important than improving one's game.

An interesting case in point to the contrary is the development of Pete Sampras. As a junior, Sampras had a good two-handed backhand, but his coach felt that he could be better if he changed to a one-handed backhand, due to his potential as a serve and volley player. He courageously made this change even though it dipped his rankings for several years. Sampras and his coach should be applauded for not being solely driven by rankings and outcome, but being more interested in long-term improvement (which would likely lead to more positive outcomes).

Performance Goals

Performance goals focus on achieving standards or performance objectives independently of other competitors, usually making comparisons with one's own previous performance. For this reason, performance goals tend to be more flexible and more importantly, within your control. In essence, success is redefined in terms of exceeding your own goal rather than merely beating an opponent. Thus, winning and losing takes a back seat to achieving a specific level of performance. This is not to say that winning is unimportant—it clearly is in our society. Rather, winning should not be the sole focus of tennis players since it is, at least in part, out of your control. The nice thing about performance goals is that they can be reached regardless of how your opponent might be playing. In fact, in several of our goal-setting studies with Division 1 athletes and Olympic athletes (including one study focusing on junior tennis players), we found that approximately 35% of the time, athletes' number one goal was to improve performance with about 25% indicating that winning was the number one goal followed by enjoyment (having fun) at 20% (Weinberg et al.,1993, 2000). So, despite the societal emphasis on winning, many athletes and tennis players had learned that focusing on improving their own performance as well as having fun, were also very important goals for them (and basically under their control). The importance of setting performance versus outcome goals is seen in the comments of Steffi Graf:

> You can't measure success if you never failed. My father has taught me that if you really want to reach your goals, you can't spend any time worrying about whether you're going to win or lose. Focus only on getting better.

Therefore, there are several benefits of setting performance goals including:

- They make you responsible for your own progress (or lack of progress).
- Your motivation and self-confidence can be built up since you are in control of your improvement.
- You can concentrate fully on the development of your own game and not worry too much about your opponent (although scouting is always useful).

Let me now provide you with some examples of performance goals. Remember that the number of goals is unlimited; the ones that you choose should be selected according to your own needs and abilities. Finally, performance goals can be set for competitive matches as well as practices. Some examples include the following:

In Competitive Matches

- Reducing my double faults from 5 per set to 2 per set
- Improving my successful passing shots from 40% to 50%
- Improving my first serve percentage from 50% to 60%
- Reducing my unforced errors to winners ratio from 2:1 to 1:1

In Practice

- Hitting 10 consecutive forehands and backhands crosscourt without missing
- Hitting 10 overheads in a row from past the service line without missing
- Hitting 10 consecutive good serves at 3/4 speed
- Hitting 15 consecutive ground strokes past the service line without missing

Process Goals

Recently, there has been a move in the sport psychology literature to recognize process goals as well performance and outcome goals. Specifically, *process goals* focus on the actions a player must engage in during performance to execute or perform well. For example a tennis player may set a goal of every stroke keeping her racquet head low (below the level of the waist) in order to impart topspin to her ground strokes. Similarly, another process goal could be tossing the ball in front of you, to land in a designated part of the court (you could draw a small circle just inside the baseline), so that you might get your body weight into the serve. Note that these goals are not related to the outcome of a particular shot (i.e., whether it went in or not). Rather, process goals are typically focused on the execution of a shot; helping provide cues as to how to hit a shot properly. As a result, most process goals tend to occur in practice sessions as this is where players should generally be working on honing the execution of their strokes. If you can reach these process goals consistently in practice, then this should lead to enhanced performance in matches. In fact, research (Kingston & Hardy, 1997) has clearly indicated that process goals can facilitate not only performance, but can help reduce a player's anxiety and build a sense of confidence.

Combining Different Types of Goals

Although each type of goal is important and can help improve your tennis performance, research (Filby, Maynard, & Graydon,1999) has revealed that a combination of different types of goals is consistently related to top performance. So it's not necessarily that one goal is better than another goal. In fact, recent research has revealed that elite athletes typically are high on setting both performance and outcome goals. So these athletes not only want to perform well, they also want to win. But it is up to you to choose the best combination of goals that fits your needs, interests, and abilities. I would recommend that process goals be mostly practice-oriented, performance goals practice and competition-oriented and outcome goals competition-oriented. The focus in competition should be on performance goals although some outcome goals could also be used as long as they don't become the main or sole focus of matches, since this can create anxiety and inappropriate thoughts or self-talk. In fact, for every outcome goal a tennis player sets, there should be several performance and process goals that would lead to achieving that outcome. Therefore, to win a particular match (outcome goal), you might need to focus in practice on keeping the racquet head low to impart more topspin (process goal), thus providing more margin for error as well as keeping your unforced errors to winners ratio down to 1:1 (performance goal).

Why Goals Work

There is a vast amount of research in the industrial/organizational literature indicating the effectiveness of goal setting on performance. In fact, there are now over 500 studies, conducted with over 50,000 participants, across 90 different tasks, in 10 different countries. But results remain very consistent, with approximately 90% of the studies finding that specific hard goals produce significantly better performance than easy goals, do your best goals or no goals (Locke & Latham, 1990). Although not nearly as longstanding or numerous, the sport psychology literature has seen a recent surge of goal-setting studies (which now number about 60) that indicate the same positive effect of goals on performance as does the industrial/organizational literature. In looking at percent improvement, it appears that on the average, setting goals can increase performance in the neighborhood of 10-15%. Wouldn't you like to improve your tennis game by 10-15%? Sometimes even a very small improvement of 1-2% can make a significant difference in a tennis player's ability and game. A point here and there can often mean the difference in a match. Before focusing on the specific principles in setting goals, let's briefly discuss why goals have such an important and consistent effect on performance.

Goals Help Prioritize What's Most Important To You

Goals can help put tennis in perspective with other aspects of your life such as social, business, personal, and academic. If improving your tennis game is really important to you, then it would receive a higher priority than say going out with your friends (see Table 4.1). Similarly, goals can help prioritize what is most important within tennis itself. For example, is it more important to work on improving your second serve or your approach shots?

Table 4.1	Prioritizing Your Goals

Research in the popular and business literatures indicates that prioritizing your goals can lead to improved productivity. Setting priorities helps you formulate more specific goals that can guide your day-to-day behavior. This exercise will help you prioritize your tennis goals to help determine what aspects of your game to focus on in practice (feel free to add on additional items that are specific to your game). So try to use the following scoring system to prioritize your tennis goals.

A = most important
B = somewhat important
C = less important

Skill	Importance Rating
Improve movement and footwork	_____
Improve first serve percentage	_____
Improve service return	_____
Improve consistency of ground strokes	_____
Improve volley	_____
Improve overhead	_____
Improve mid court game	_____
Improve slice backhand	_____
Improve crosscourt forehand	_____
Improve mental toughness	_____
Improve concentration on every point	_____

Priorities of A, B, and C, for example, could be used to help you determine what is most important for you and what areas of your life (or your game) you need to be working on.

Goals Provide Direction and Focus Attention

Goals can help direct your attention to important elements of playing tennis, which you may not ordinarily have attended to in the past. When you set a goal, it helps you stay focused on a course of action to achieve that goal. For example, one of the junior tennis players I worked with knew that his volleys needed to be improved, but he never really got around to hitting many volleys in practice because he preferred to pound ground strokes. So we set a goal to improve the consistency of his volleys by working on volleys for 20 minutes each practice, followed up with more specific process and performance goals. As a result, this player started to focus on improving his volley as part of his practice regimen.

This eventually led to building his confidence in his volleying skills and using the volley successfully more often in competitive matches.

Goals Increase Effort and Persistence

When you set a goal for yourself that is important, you will generally put forth effort to achieve that goal. You might want to set a goal to win your club championship, which comes up in three months. This outcome goal would have to be supported by some process and performance goals to help make this a reality. Therefore, you would typically try hard to reach your performance and process goals, which might involve improving your passing shots and overhead smash. In any case, your goals would help you keep striving and working hard both in practice and competition.

Goals Maintain Motivation

Without goals, practicing can become boring and less meaningful, resulting in a loss of desire and motivation. However, tennis players are only able to reach their potential if they are motivated. Although most of us are motivated from time to time (maybe when there is a big tournament ahead), goals help us to sustain motivation over a longer period of time. Players who have short-and long-term goals (discussed later in this chapter) understand that the drudgery and fatigue that sometimes accompany practice, will result in successful performance in the weeks, months and even years ahead. Therefore, goals are important to help show the connection between your day-to-day behaviors and your future performances.

Goals Increase Learning

Setting goals also promotes searching for effective ways of accomplishing these goals. In essence, it's not enough just to set a goal, but you have to figure out how to reach the goal. In using another example from my work with tennis players, there was one junior player who wanted to improve her second serve in terms of pace and "kick." So I asked her how she should go about doing this? Using her feedback, we agreed that she needed to speed up (not slow down) her swing as well as toss the ball further behind her to impart the proper topspin (which increases one's margin of error). So she set some process goals in these areas and devoted 20 minutes each practice to improving her second serve. Over the next couple of months, according to her coach's assessment, her second serve definitely improved in speed and "kick."

Identify Your Goals

Before we discuss principles of how to set goals, you should first identify what it is that you want to achieve. Younger players in particular need to sort out their own goals from the goals of their parents and coach (although their input is certainly important). In helping you determine your goals, you might ask yourself some questions regarding your tennis, like the ones provided below.

- What strokes need the most improvement?
- What are my greatest strengths?
- What type of player do I want to be in 6 months? In one year?
- What is my physical condition?
- Do I understand strategy and tactics?
- How much time am I willing to put into practice?
- What are the most enjoyable aspects of tennis?
- What do I like least about playing competitive tennis?

Thinking about the answers to these questions should help you crystallize your thinking regarding what it is that you need to focus on in your tennis game. After you identify the areas in which to set your goals, you are ready to apply the principles of effective goal setting.

Goal-Setting Principles

By this time, I hope you feel that goals can help your tennis game (and other areas of your life). However, our research (Weinberg & Gould, 1999) has clearly indicated that not all goals are equally effective in improving performance and enhancing psychological well-being. So it is important that you follow the goal-setting guidelines provided below, to maximize the benefits of setting goals.

Set Challenging, Realistic Goals

One of the key principles of achieving optimal performance and getting "in the zone" is having a match between skills and challenges. This could, in large part, be accomplished through setting goals that are challenging, but yet realistically attainable, if you put forth consistent effort. In addition, one of the strongest findings in the goal-setting literature is that goals need to be moderately difficult and challenging. Goals are of little value if little effort is needed to achieve them (we become satisfied with less), or if they are so difficult that they produce consistent failure, leading to frustration and reduced confidence.

Therefore, the secret is to strike a balance between goal challenge and achievability, which is no easy task. The more experience a player or a coach has, the better able they will be at finding this delicate balance. So if a junior player is ranked 25th in his section, then becoming number 3 by the end of the year would seem unrealistic. But one has to be careful in determining what is realistic. In essence, it's okay to shoot for the stars and want to turn professional one day, as this dream will come true for a select few. However, you need to separate your dreams from reality. So keep your dreams (and even have a dream goal— see Table 4.2) but make sure you set some challenging goals in the present, that might make it possible to achieve these dreams in the future.

Table 4.2	Setting Your Goals

1. Dream Goal (Long-Term). What is potentially possible in the long-term if you stretch all of your limits?

_____

_____

1. Dream Goal (This Year). What is potentially possible if all of your limits are stretched this year?

_____

_____

3. Realistic Long-Term Goal (This Year). What do you feel is a realistic performance goal that you can achieve this year based on your current skills, potential for improvement, and motivation?

_____

_____

4. This realistic performance goal can be broken down into short-term goals such as
   a) Monthly Goals_____
   b) Weekly Goals_____
   c) Daily Goals_____

5. Strategies for Achieving Goals (as well as barriers) in
   a) Daily Practice _____
   b) Match Competition_____

Repeat the above for additional Long-Term Goals

Set Specific Measurable Goals

Research has strongly indicated that specific, measurable goals affect behavioral change and increase performance more effectively than general "do your best" goals. Unfortunately, many players and coaches still set goals in fairly general terms, such as wanting to improve their consistency from the baseline, become more mentally tough, or reducing their unforced errors. While all of these may be worthwhile goals, in their present form, they are not very useful or informative.

For example, what does becoming more mentally tough really mean? Does it mean to improve concentration, deal better with adversity, improve your confidence, or not being disturbed by bad line calls? Similarly, what does reduce unforced errors mean? Does it mean hitting the ball with more topspin, hitting the ball more in the middle of the court, or hitting the ball at 3/4 pace? As you can tell, without clearly specifying your goals in measurable terms, you become hard-pressed to know when and if you have reached your goal.

Let's take reducing unforced errors as an example. A more specific goal might be to reduce the ratio between unforced errors and winners from 2:1 to 1:1 by hitting with more topspin. Thus, you are not trying to hit more winners, but rather simply reducing your errors. A coach can monitor the unforced error/winner ratio in a match (performance goal) and note whether you were using topspin whenever possible (process goal). After a number of opportunities, if you didn't achieve your goal because you were still hitting the ball close to the line, you might practice hitting the ball more in the middle of the court. You could mark the court during practice and set goals for hitting the ball a certain amount of times (e.g.,15 out of 20) inside the designated areas (let's say three feet from each sideline). In summary, be precise, state your goals in measurable terms, specify the behaviors you want to perform, and set a target date to reach your goals. As up-and-coming star Andy Roddick recently said, *"Things seem to come easier if I have a clear goal, and not just in tennis. For example, I set a goal not to have to qualify for the French Open in 2001, and I reached that goal with some good wins in the preceding months."*

Set Short- and Long-Term Goals

It takes time to make changes in one's tennis game. To achieve positive results down the road, we need both short- and long-term goals. However, when I ask tennis players their goals, they usually identify long-term objectives such as getting a college scholarship in tennis, achieving a certain state ranking at the end of the year, or winning the club championship. But to achieve these long-term goals usually requires setting and meeting short-term goals.

One way to think about the relationship of short- and long-term goals is to think of a staircase with the long-term (or dream) goal at the top, the present level of ability at the bottom step, and a sequence of progressively linked, short-term goals connecting the top and bottom of the stairs. For example, with one player I worked with, her long-term goal was to be ranked in the top 5 in her state in the next age division (she was currently number 25 in the 16s and wanted a top 5 finish in the 18s). To achieve this, she set short-term outcome goals of moving up from number 25 in first year 16s to number 10 in 2nd year 16s. For first year in the 18s her goal was to be number 10 and for second year it was to be number 5. To accomplish this ranking, she also set specific short-term performance and process goals such as improving her first serve percentage from 50% to 60%, reducing her unforced errors in matches by 25%, and making sure she extended her arms when hitting her two-handed backhand. Thus, what appeared to be a daunting task, became much more possible with these short-term goals (many of which were daily goals) to focus on accomplishing (she wound up 3rd in the 18s). Table 4.3 provides an example of setting short-and long-term goals.

Therefore, short-term goals are important. They not only provide you with feedback regarding how you are progressing toward your long-term goal, but also help keep you motivated because you can see immediate improvements in performance. As a result, of the feedback you get from your short-term goals, if it appears that you will easily reach your long-term goal or possibly never reach it, you could then reevaluate and change your long-term goal. For example, if your goal was to play number 2 on your college team as a junior and you are number 10 as a sophomore, then maybe you need to lower your goal to making the top 6. But if you are already number 2 as a sophomore, then maybe you might want to be number 1 as a junior. In either case, motivation would be maximized since your goal is now more challenging.

Identify Specific Plans to Reach Goals

As noted earlier, one of the key reasons that goals work is that they can provide strategies for reaching goals. Unfortunately, I have seen many tennis players set goals without having any strategies for reaching their goals. So although you might know that you want to get to Los Angeles from New York, you then have to map out exactly what highways you are going to take to get there. Similarly, in tennis, let's say that one of your goals is to reduce your unforced errors in each set from 15 to 10 within the next month. This is a specific measurable goal but how would you accomplish it? In essence, what would be your strategy for reaching this goal? Some possibilities include: (a) hitting with more topspin to increase your margin of error; (b) shortening your backswing to avoid over-hitting; (c) hitting more balls cross court since the net is lower and there is more room to hit than down the line; and (d) devoting 15 minutes of each practice to just working on the consistency of your ground strokes. These are just examples, but the point is that you need to devise a strategy (or strategies) that you can implement to help meet your goal. Andre Agassi has his own way of setting specific goals and plans each day. *Every morning, when I wake up, the first thing I do is look in the mirror and ask "what is it that I want to do, and what is it that I need to work on today."*

Write Down Your Goals

In our research with both tennis coaches and athletes (Weinberg, Burke, & Jackson, 1997; Weinberg, Butt, & Knight, 2001; Weinberg, Butt, Knight, & Perritt, 2001); we consistently found that both coaches and athletes did not systematically write down and record their goals. This is despite the fact that research clearly shows that writing goals down increases a person's commitment to the goal while at the same time helping keep goals in the forefront, instead of fading away. Goals mean nothing unless you are committed to them and have a permanent record of them, including their progress. In addition, goals help ensure commitment, effort and persistence.

Table 4.3	Short- and Long-Term Goals

Directions: Determine a long-term goal toward which you are striving (I will give an example of winning the club championship next year—you came in third last year). In the space provided below, list three or four progressively more challenging goals that will move you toward achieving your long-term goal.

Win the club championship
Long-Term Goal

Hit 20 ground strokes in a row past the service line
Goal 3

Hit 10 backhands in a row past the service line
Goal 2

Hit 10 forehands in a row in the court during practice
Goal 1

Finished 3rd due to baseline inconsistency
Current Performance

Long-Term Goal

Goal 3

Goal 2

Goal 1

Current Performance

Set Practice and Competition Goals

In my experience, many tennis players and coaches make the mistake of setting goals predominantly or solely for competition. As noted earlier, goals (especially process goals) should also be set for practice. Like many other sports, tennis players practice much more than they actually play competitive (tournament) matches. But do you really practice or do you just hit some balls with a friend and say "let's play?" Similarly, do you go through practice without ever really focusing on a particular shot or part of your game such as just hit for an hour with no real focus or plan?

Practice can certainly be boring but it can be "jazzed up" by setting process and performance goals. These goals can provide added motivation and direction for what you need to accomplish. For example, how many players work on their approach shots? This is a difficult shot, which balances depth and speed versus accuracy, but yet it is not practiced often. When we get in a match we wonder why we are not hitting our approach shot well or are even afraid to hit it, since we lack confidence in this stroke (not surprising since we rarely practice it). So what if we set a goal of hitting 5 approach shots in a row within 3 feet of the baseline (we'd draw a line on the court 3 feet from the baseline) to emphasize depth on our approach shot. First of all, you should be more focused on your approach shot and paying attention to hitting it properly. Second, as you get 3 or 4 in a row, the pressure mounts (you don't want to start all over again) so you might get tight like you would in a match. In essence, you might start actually feeling like you would in a competitive event and thus this could act as simulation training.

Provide Goal Support

It is sometimes tough to stay on course and stay focused on achieving your goals. One of the ways research has clearly shown to help individuals achieve their goals is for others to provide support for these goals. These others could be friends, family members, coaches, or teammates. For young tennis players, parental support is particularly important since parents are central in the developing lives of young tennis players. Asking players about their goals and providing emotional support is critical. But parents and coaches alike should support the process and performance goals set by young tennis players and not focus solely on outcome. This support will allow young players to continue to improve their games and not get too caught up with rankings or won-loss records.

For adults, research has been very consistent in indicating that spousal or significant other support is one of the most effective ways of helping loved ones reach their goals. Support does not mean you are not critical of mistakes or lack of effort. Rather, it means trying to stay positive and help build up, rather than tear down players by giving them instructional, positive feedback that can help them improve and reach their goals. To see if you have a good understanding of the principles of goal setting just discussed, complete the exercise in Table 4.4.

Table 4.4	**Analyzing Your Goals**

Instructions: List three of your goals for tennis

#1 _____

#2 _____

#3 _____

Goal-Setting Principles: Rate each of your goals on the five principles listed below by placing a checkmark in the appropriate column if your goal conforms to that principle.

	Performance	**Realistic**	**Specific**	**Measurable**	**Action Plan**
#1	_____	_____	_____	_____	_____
#2	_____	_____	_____	_____	_____
#3	_____	_____	_____	_____	_____

Based on the above analysis what are your goal-setting strengths and weaknesses?

Strengths:

_____

_____

Weaknesses:

_____

_____

Instructions: Below are three general goals. After each one, write two specific, measurable goals (e.g., hit 65% of first serves), that lead to reaching the general goal. Then in the space below (number 4) specify one general goal that you have and two specific goals to reach it.

1. To improve my serve

    a. _____

    b. _____

2. To improve my baseline consistency

    a. _____

    b. _____

3. To improve my mental toughness

    a. _____

    b. _____

4. _____

    a. _____

    b. _____

A Goal-Setting System for Coaches

Hopefully you are now well versed in the principles of goal setting and realize that there is a scientific method for making goals more effective. Those of you who teach or coach tennis might be asking, "How can I implement a goal setting program with my team or at my club?" Although there are many different goal-setting systems, most of them include three different stages: (a) Preparation and Planning; (b) Education and Acquisition; and (c) Implementation and Follow-Up.

Preparation and Planning Phase

As a coach, you do not want to enter the season unprepared and thus considerable thought and preparation regarding goals must precede the actual season. The time spent on preparing the goal-setting process saves hours of work once the program is implemented. Here are the things you need to do to prepare and plan.

Assess Abilities and Needs

The first step would be to start thinking about identifying some specific team and individual needs based on the abilities of the players. For example, some of your needs might include physical conditioning, development of fundamentals (e.g., strokes) sportsmanship, improvement of mental skills, and footwork.

Set Goals in Diverse Areas

Once you identify your specific needs, the next step is to turn these needs into specific goals. It is important that goals be set in a variety of areas as noted above, such as enjoyment, psychological skills, sportsmanship, fitness, and playing time, instead of focusing only on performance. Remember that players participate in tennis for a variety of reasons (including affiliation, fun, and skill improvement) and therefore you should have goals set in diverse areas so everyone can feel successful. In essence, goals need to be relevant to players' needs and thus it is important that you understand their commitment and psychological make-up.

Plan Goal Achievement Strategies

As discussed previously, strategies must be planned that players can use to achieve their goals. Without specific strategies, players are likely to fall short in achieving their goals because they don't know how to go about reaching them. Therefore, you need to do your homework before meeting with your team or individual players, having specific strategies worked out to meet specific goals. Of course, you can solicit input from the players, but you should be ready to offer specific suggestions regarding goal strategies.

Education and Acquisition Phase

Once the preparation and planning phase has been completed, you can begin educating your players on the most effective ways to set goals. This involves setting up some meetings where specific goal-setting information is imparted.

Schedule Initial Meeting

A formal meeting at the beginning of the season is a good place to start. Here, basic information concerning goal setting can be given such as goal specificity, short- and long-term goals, process, performance, and outcome goals, etc. In this meeting, players could be asked to identify effective and ineffective goals. But don't have your players set their goals at this meeting. Rather, have them think about specific areas in which they can set goals, and be prepared to come to the next meeting with specific goals in mind. In this way, players will have the opportunity to think about and consider what their goals should be.

Follow-Up Team and Individual Meetings

A second team meeting should be scheduled shortly after the first one to discuss the goals that players' were formulating during the past several days. Discuss these team goals in light of the principles of goal-setting you provided the team during the initial meeting. Through discussion and consensus, team goals should be established and specific strategies identified for reaching these goals.

It is generally a good idea to set up one-on-one meetings with players to discuss their specific individual goals. These meetings could be brief (10-15 minutes) and focus on using the goal strategies identified to help set goals in specific areas. Always try to involve players in setting these goals so that commitment is maximized. These goals should be recorded along with strategies to achieve them and put in a place where the player will see them every day. Some coaches post them on a bulletin board or have players post them on their lockers. Whatever way you choose to record and illustrate team and individual goals, make sure that these goals remain important and a high priority for the players to accomplish.

Implementation and Follow-Up Phase

Once players have learned to set goals, then you need to carefully monitor how players are doing in relation to these goals. In essence, goal evaluation is critical.

Identify Goal Evaluation Procedures

Evaluation is typically the final phase of any goal-setting program. Unfortunately, this is often neglected as coaches get involved in the season and either fall behind or totally forget the evaluation of goals. So anticipate when you will be busy and estimate how much time you will have available for goal evaluation and follow-up. Many coaches streamline the evaluation process by having managers keep and post relevant practice and match statistics related to players' goals.

Plan for Goal Reevaluation

One way to ensure that at least some evaluation takes place is to schedule goal evaluation meetings periodically throughout the season. This is a good time to discuss the progress that players and the team as a whole are making toward achieving their goals. Since goal-setting is not a perfect science, it is entirely possible that players may have already reached the goals set or may be far away (possibly due to injury) from achieving their goals. For example, a player may have set a goal to reach 60% of first serves after the first five matches. Maybe she already exceeded this goal (i.e., has a 62% first serve percentage) and therefore needs to up her goal to 65%. Whether goals are increased or decreased, the coach needs to provide players with specific feedback concerning the progress they are making toward achieving their goals. If you provide feedback in written form (e.g., match statistics, your own evaluation of improvement in a particular area), then this will enhance motivation. It is important to follow-through on your goal-setting program with evaluations; this shows your commitment and dedication toward the program and achieving the goals that are set. Your personal involvement and social support will provide a model for your players to follow and maximize the effectiveness of your goal-setting program.

CHAPTER 5

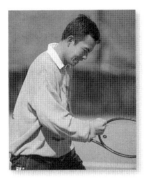

CONFIDENCE

The whole thing is never to get negative about yourself. Sure it's possible that the other guy you're playing is tough, and that he may have beaten you the last time you played, and okay, maybe you haven't been playing all that well yourself. But the minute you start thinking about these things you're dead. I go out to every match convinced that I'm going to win, That's all there is to it.

(Tarshis, 1977, p. 102)
Jimmy Connors (before playing Bjorn Borg in the finals of the US Open)

The difference between me at my peak and me in the last few years of my career is that when I was the champion I had the ultimate in confidence. I could almost make myself hit that shot when it mattered most.

Billy Jean King

After a really tough, high-level three-set match against Patrick Rafter, Marat Safin had this to say about confidence:

When the week started, I had no confidence. I'm not going to say I'm going to win the US Open now, but I do feel confident and I feel it's all coming together.

Moving out of the world of tennis for a moment, the quote by automobile developer, Henry Ford speaks directly to the effect of confidence on behavior.

Whether you think you can or think you can't, you are right.

The above comments capture the critical role that confidence can play in a tennis player's mental outlook and ultimate success. You should remember from Chapter 2, that self-confidence was one of the psychological states consistently related to peak performance and being "in the zone." Research has clearly demonstrated that the most consistent factor distinguishing highly successful from less successful athletes (including tennis players) is confidence. Furthermore, in interviews with top tennis players, they consistently refer to confidence as a key factor in their success. Or conversely, they talk about not having confidence, or having self-doubts, which typically undermine performance. So it appears obvious that players need to develop and maintain their self-confidence if they want to be successful and play their best. But before, I talk about how to build confidence, let's take a closer look at exactly what it is, since this will provide clues for how to build it.

Defining Self-Confidence

Although tennis players often say "I really have confidence in my serve," or "I just felt confident in my ability to come back from behind," or "I felt so confident that every shot was going in," what is it that they really mean? In defining confidence, sport psychologists simply refer to it as the belief that you can successfully perform a desired behavior. In essence, *it is believing that you possess the skills and abilities to be successful.* These skills or abilities in tennis might be stroke related like believing in your serve and volley (Patrick Rafter), return of serve (Andre Agassi), backhand (Venus Williams), or forehand (Steffi Graf). Or they might be related to some of your mental skills like your ability to concentrate, ability to hit the right shot at the right time, ability to cope with pressure, or ability to come from behind.

The common factor in all of these is simply your belief that you can perform that particular skill or behavior. Confident tennis players expect to be successful and believe in their capacity to perform the actions necessary to be successful and win matches. So it's not just a matter of stroke production; confident tennis players believe that they can figure out the proper strategies to win matches and have the mental skills to play well. However, sometimes players lack confidence, doubt themselves at important points in matches, and simply expect to lose. These doubts and negative expectations can really undermine a player's performance, as we will see in the next section.

Undermining Confidence—Placing Limits on Ourselves

When you doubt your ability to succeed or expect something to go wrong, you are creating what is called a negative self-fulfilling prophesy—which means that expecting something to happen actually helps cause it to happen. Unfortunately, this phenomenon is all too common in tennis players. Negative self-fulfilling prophesies are psychological barriers that lead to a vicious cycle. Specifically, players expect to fail. This expectation, in part, causes them to fail, which lowers their self-image and confidence, thus increasing expectations of future failure. For example, after you lose to a player several times in a row, you then start to believe that you can't beat this player. In turn, your confidence and motivation get lower, which leads to actual poor performance in the future against this player and, of course, continued failure.

But things don't have to be this way, as seen in this comment by former top 10 player Vitas Geralitis after losing to Bjorn Borg 16 times in a row. After playing a great match and finally beating Borg on the17th attempt, Geralitis (who was known to have a good sense of humor) took the microphone from the commentator at the start of a post match interview, and stat-ed *"nobody, but nobody, beats Vitas Geralitis 17 times in a row."* Although somewhat kidding, Geralitis went on to say that it was very difficult keeping up his confidence against Borg after so many losses. But he knew that he played Borg tough on several occasions (including a very tough and spirited loss at Wimbledon, 8-6 in the 5th set) and felt that if he played well he could beat Borg. Therefore, he said he maintained his confidence, despite so many losses in a row to Borg. Without keeping his confidence, Geralitis felt he would never have beaten Borg.

A classical example of someone overcoming a negative self-fulfilling prophesy, is the story of how Roger Bannister broke the 4-minute mile. Before 1954, several runners were timed at 4:03, 4:02, and 4:01, but nobody could crack the four-minute barrier. In fact, a well-known physiologist claimed that it was physically impossible to run a mile in under four minutes. This created a negative self-fulfilling prophesy among many runners, but not for Roger Bannister. He had stated that the four-minute mile was most definitely possible, under the right conditions. He created these conditions, and in fact broke the four-minute mile in a very courageous effort. Bannister's feat was impressive, but what's really interesting is that about a dozen runners broke the record in the next year. Why? Did everyone suddenly get faster or start training harder? Of course not. What happened was that runners finally believed it could be done. Until Roger Bannister broke the barrier, runners had been placing psychological lim-its on themselves, because they felt it just wasn't possible to break the four-minute mile.

These same types of results have been found with coaches and teachers. That is, they often create expectations regarding how well they think their athletes or students will per-form. In most cases, performers then will perform up to the level of expectations of their coaches and teachers (whether these expectations are positive or negative). For example, I worked with a junior tennis player who was consistently told by her coaches that she would never amount to anything without a stronger second serve. In fact, her serve was constantly criticized for being too unreliable in pressure situations. And sure enough she doubted her second serve abilities and tended to double-fault when the match got tough and pressure got high. We worked on keeping up her confidence and just staying positive on her second serve (we didn't touch mechanics). With a stronger belief in her second serve, her first serve also actually improved since she wasn't always worried about what would happen if she missed her first serve. She improved her second serve greatly over the ensuing months and would rarely double fault at critical times in a match. This helped her gain a college scholarship and continue four years of successful college tennis.

Your belief (or doubt) in yourself can be very temporary or it can get to be a pattern of the way you think about yourself and your tennis game. Keeping up your confidence and believing in yourself is highlighted in the following comment by all-time great Rod Laver:

> You get into winning or losing patterns. A lot of it is getting the breaks. If you win a lot of close matches, your attitude when you get into close matches is, "No sweat, I've been here before and I'll be here again." But if you start to lose a lot of close ones, and you get ahead in a match, you start to think, "Oh, oh, here it comes again."
>
> (Tarshis, 1977, p. 94)

Similarly, keeping up one's confidence is highlighted by these comments by John McEnroe.

> I'm confident on the court. I like the way I play. I have no particular weakness. I think it's the mark of great players to be confident in tough situations.

Benefits of Confidence

We have alluded to the importance of confidence in enhancing performance and producing positive behavior change. But now let's briefly look at the specific benefits that high levels of self-confidence, can have on tennis players.

Confidence Increases Effort

Our research has consistently shown that how much effort and persistence players put forth in pursuit of their tennis goals depends largely on their self-confidence. This becomes especially important in that many tennis matches are played against opponents of reasonably equal ability. The one who puts forth more effort, in this case, is the one who will usually win.

Confidence Affects Goals

Confident players usually set challenging goals and pursue them actively. We know from Chapter 2 that challenging goals help skills match challenges, thus making getting in the zone more probable. In addition, as seen in Chapter 4, challenging goals is one of the keys to successful goal-setting. So confident players, by setting challenging goals, are maximizing motivation and commitment as well as performance. For example, if you are a 3.0 player (sort of a beginner), then it would probably not be realistic to set a goal to have more winners than unforced errors in your matches since it would typically lead to frustration and failure. Conversely, a 5.0 player (very solid player) setting a service goal of making 40% of his first serves, would probably find this too easy and motivation and commitment would be lost.

Confidence Facilitates Concentration

When you feel confident, your mind is free to focus on the task at hand. You can play almost on "automatic pilot" without being slowed down by worries or distracting thoughts. When you lack confidence in tennis, you tend to worry about a missed shot, missed opportunity, or what others think about you. These potential distractions to your concentration will be discussed in Chapter 8.

Confidence Arouses Positive Emotions

Research has clearly revealed that when you feel confident, you are more likely to remain calm and relaxed under pressure. This state of mind also allows you to be assertive and aggressive at key moments in a match. So even though it might be late in the third set, if you are confident, you are relaxed enough to go for your shots and not get tight.

Confidence Affects Game Strategies

We know that at times, tennis players play "not to lose" instead of "playing to win." These phrases sound similar but they produce very different styles of play. And as we know too well, many tennis matches come down to shot selection on critical points. It's not unusual to find players pushing the ball on important points, hoping their opponent will make an error. Players lacking confidence, in essence, just don't want to make a mistake. Or conversely, to relieve the pressure of an important point, other players will "overhit" and go for low percentage, ill-advised shots just to get the point over. But the confident player takes normal swings and stays relaxed, making good decisions under pressure. Andre Agassi (at least in his later years) is a good example of a confident player, hitting out on big points, but still leaving some margin for error. It's this balance between errors and winners that becomes so important on critical points.

Confidence Affects Psychological Momentum

Anyone who has played tennis, knows that oftentimes, it is a game of momentum with each player winning several games in a row or having two lopsided sets such as 6-1, 1-6. Sometimes momentum can change on one shot, such as in a tiebreaker. Other times it might be a contested line call or missing an opportunity for a break of serve. Then again it may build up gradually over a few games. In any case, at the core of shifts in momentum is the ever present self-confidence. A match between Pete Sampras and Patrick Rafter at the 2000 Wimbledon makes a good case for momentum and confidence. Rafter led one set to love and was up 4-1 in the tiebreaker with two serves coming. But Sampras managed to return serve well and win those points and then he never looked back, winning that tiebreaker and the final two sets rather handily. As Sampras noted after the match, *the momentum really shifted on those two points in the tiebreaker, after I won those my confidence returned and I was able to go for my shots.*

The tennis scoring system also makes for momentum shifts and confidence changes. In a U.S. Open semifinal match, Guillermo Vilas was leading Manual Orantes, 2 sets to zero and up 5-1 in the third, when Orantes made a miraculous comeback to win in 5 sets (he went on to beat Jimmy Connors in the finals the next day). As Orantes crawled back into the match, momentum shifted slowly, but time was not going to run out on Orantes. As Orantes noted, *after every game that I won, I gained a little more confidence. At first I didn't really believe I could come back from so far behind to win. But then as I won a few games I started to believe. I knew that time was not going to run out on me.*

These observations were interesting, so my colleagues and I conducted a series of studies investigating, coming from behind in tennis matches after losing the first set (Ranson & Weinberg, 1985). Looking at approximately 20,000 USTA (juniors and collegiate) matches, we found that the winners of the first set (in the best 2 of 3 set matches) usually had momentum and won their matches approximately 90% of the time (this was true a little more often for males then females). But then we looked at over 500 professional matches, and found that the top 20 ranked players in the world were able to come back to win about 37% of the time (much more than players of high, but somewhat lesser ability).

The question becomes, why are these top players able to come back and win much more often than other talented players? The answer appears to lie in the elusive concept of confidence. Of course the top 20 players have great physical talent, but then again, so do many other top players. Our studies have revealed, however, that one of the most consistent differences that separate the top players from the rest of the field is their belief in their own abilities. Thus after losing the first set, top players see the situation as a challenge (remember the skill-challenge balance from Chapter 2), and usually put forth more effort and determination to try to win the match. In essence, confident players never give up until the final point is lost, and the great champions rarely, if ever, lose their confidence (the notion of psychological momentum will be discussed in more detail in Chapter 11).

Sources of Confidence

Before we discuss how confidence affects performance, it would be important to understand where one gets confidence in the first place. Fortunately some recent research (see Vealey, 2001 for a review) has systematically assessed athletes' sources of confidence and these are summarized in Table 5.1. It appears that the strongest sense of confidence comes from actual accomplishments in sport whether they indicate personal improvement, usually through practice and drilling (mastery), or through beating people in competitions (demonstration of ability). Such was the case in the comments of Sebastian Grosjean before playing (and eventually beating) Yevgeny Kafelnikov in the year-end 2001 Masters Cup. *For the past three weeks I have been playing great tennis, so I'm really confident for today.*

Physical / mental preparation was also a highly valued source of confidence and this can be best seen in the preparation of Andre Agassi. When he was nearly to 30 years old (old in the professional tennis world) he started to work more and more on his preparation for

Table 5.1 Sources of Sport Confidence

Source	Confidence Derived from...
Mastery	Mastering or improving personal skills
Demonstration of Ability	Demonstrating more ability than an opponent
Physical/Mental Preparation	Feeling physically and mentally prepared to perform
Physical Self-Presentation	Perceptions of one's physical self (how one looks)
Social Support	Perceiving encouragement from significant others
Vicarious Experience	Watching others, like teammates, perform successfully
Coach's Leadership	Believing coach is skilled in decision-making
Environmental Comfort	Feeling comfortable in a competitive environment
Situational Favorableness	Feeling that the breaks of the situation are in your favor

matches, especially working hard on his physical conditioning, to put him (by his own admission) in the best shape of his life, Agassi has often said that this conditioning has given him confidence that he could stay on the court as long as it took to win a match. In essence, he felt that he was in better condition to play long points and long arduous matches than his opponents. So instead of simply going for winners (like he did earlier in his career), he became more exacting and hit with a greater margin of error, forcing his opponents to run longer and having the points go longer. This helped him win the French Open (giving him wins in all Grand Slams –the only current player at the time to do so) and become ranked number one in the world. Jim Courier, who retired in 1998, was also known as a player who was always physically and mentally ready to play. He may not have been the most talented player on the tour, but nobody outworked Courier in preparing for matches. This gave great confidence to his game, as Courier felt confident he could outlast you on the court both physically and mentally.

Notice, however, that the sources of sport confidence are very varied. Besides coming directly from performance accomplishments and preparation, it also emanates from several different areas. For example, we get confidence through significant others in the form of social support (especially important for female athletes), through watching others perform well, through how the coach treats us (e.g., feedback, strategy), as well as how comfortable we feel in a particular environment (e.g., clay, grass, hard courts). In studies we conducted with tennis coaches (Weinberg, Grove, & Jackson, 1992; Weinberg & Jackson, 1990), we found the top five strategies (both in terms of frequency and effectiveness) that tennis coaches used to promote confidence in their players were (a) performance improvements through drilling and instruction, (b) encouraging positive self-talk from the player, (c) liberally using rewarding statements, (d) verbally persuading the player that he or she could do it, and (e) acting confident yourself. These all relate to the sources of confidence noted above and are specific to tennis. Therefore, it is important from either a coaching or playing perspective to understand from where confidence is derived on the tennis court. This can help structure activities to maximize the sources of confidence or use some sources, which might have been underused in the past.

Confidence and Performance

Up until now, we have discussed different aspects of confidence and its importance to performance, but have not directly presented the confidence-performance relationship. It is important to note that tennis players' sense of confidence must be based on their ability level. In essence, confidence alone without the requisite ability will only get you so far. We'll discuss this in a little more depth when we talk about overconfidence. But sometimes just one important victory can boost your confidence immensely. Take Gustavo Kuerten who was a relative unknown until he won the French Open in 1998. Since then, to date, he has won two more French Opens and had risen to number one in the world ranking. That first Grand Slam win, in which he beat several top clay court players, boosted his confidence greatly, and after that he felt that he could compete with the top players. In addition, he also worked hard on his hard court game to become a more well-rounded player.

When directly looking at the confidence-performance relationship (see Figure 5.1), we see an inverted-U relationship (although a little skewed to the right). In essence, performance will increase as confidence increases up to an optimal point, whereupon further increases in confidence will produce a decrease in performance. At the top of the inverted –U, then, is optimal self-confidence. At this point you feel that you are convinced you can achieve your goals and that you will strive hard to do so. It does not necessarily mean that you will perform well, but it is essential for you to reach your potential. You can expect to make some errors and bad decisions, and you might even lose concentration occasionally. But a strong belief in yourself will help you deal with errors and mistakes effectively and keep you striving toward success. Of course, if there is an optimal level of self-confidence then we can either have too little or too much of it.

Lack of Confidence

When speaking about confidence, players who are not optimally confident usually have low levels of confidence (even though, at times, their skill level is high). It is difficult to know if a lack of confidence caused poor performance or whether poor performance caused lack of confidence. Although the answer to this question is difficult, we do know that success is never certain but self-doubt, low expectations, and lack of confidence almost assures failure. In addition, we have noted the many benefits of confidence earlier in the chapter, but there are also many drawbacks to not having confidence such as needless worry, a tendency to give up (especially in the face of adversity), focusing on mistakes, being tentative, and heightened anxiety. This sort of circular relationship between confidence and performance is emphasized by the comments of a top collegiate player.

Figure 5.1

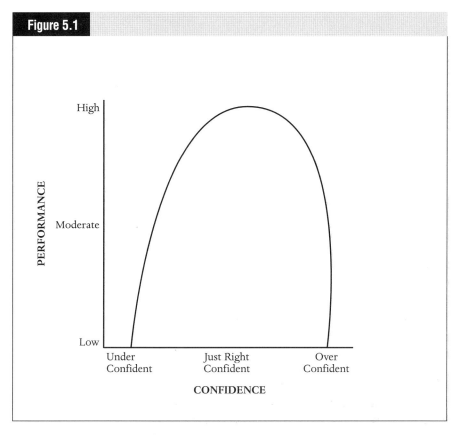

Confidence comes from hours and days and weeks and years of constant work and dedication. It's just a circle. Work and confidence, then more work and more confidence.

However, confidence could be fragile and change in an instant. For example, how many times have you seen players warm up great, hitting beautiful ground strokes, crisp volleys and cannonball serves. But once the match starts they begin pushing the ball and you never see those wonderful strokes (or if you do see them, the ball does not go consistently onto the court). Similarly, many tennis players look great for a set and a half and are rolling with confidence, But sometimes, just one missed shot (especially if it's important like a potential break of serve) may lead to a sharp drop-off in confidence and performance, as now shots are sprayed all over the place instead of the accurate placement occurring up until then. Confidence (or lack of it) is aptly summarized by the comments of Brian Gottfried, a former top 10 professional player.

The difference between feeling confident when you're playing and not feeling confident is that you never hesitate to go for your shots and you're not giving your opponents the extra opportunities you give them when you're not confident and you're trying to just keep the ball in play.

(Tarshis, 1977, p. 91)

Sometimes your confidence might be tied to a particular stroke. For example, when Goran Ivanisevic is serving well and has confidence in his serve he can be awfully tough to beat. But when his confidence and serve falters, he can quickly "go away." In fact, Julie Anthony, former professional player turned sport psychologist has argued that men generally have more confidence than women because of their bigger serves. Specifically, she stated:

I think there are more genuinely confident men players than women players because a lot of men players have tremendous confidence in their serves So when the serve is working, they figure the worst they can do is stay even. Most women don't have that luxury.

(Tarshis, 1977, p. 92)

Other times your confidence might be tied to your ability to come back from behind. So you try harder and keep focused even though you might be losing a match. But if a player lost several close matches, they may lack confidence when the match is tight into the third set. The common denominator is that when you lack confidence in your abilities as a tennis player, your game is very likely to go downhill very quickly.

Overconfidence

Although not as much of a problem as lack of confidence, overconfidence can still produce some devastating results in a player's performance. This is a tough balance act at times, as some players appears to be arrogant and cocky and some people might consider them overconfident. But the key thing with overconfidence is that it is really a sense of false confidence. In essence, when you feel that your abilities are really greater than they are (or you underestimate the abilities of your opponent) you really have a false sense of confidence. This sense of overconfidence is reflected in the comment by Bobby Riggs, after his classic match with Billie Jean King.

It was mainly a case of overconfidence on my part. I overestimated myself, and I underestimated Billie Jean's ability to meet the pressure. I let her pick the surface and the ball because I figured it wouldn't make any difference, that she would beat herself. Even when she won the first set, I wasn't worried. In fact, I tried to bet more money on myself. But I miscalculated. I ran out of gas. She started playing better and better. I started playing worse. I tried to slow up the game to keep her back but she kept the pressure on.

(Tarshis, 1977, p. 148)

This type of scenario is often repeated when players of different abilities play against one another. The better player sometimes does not come prepared to play and has a false sense of confidence (false because they were not bringing their "A" game to the court). This overconfidence often leads to early lackadaisical play by the better player, which in turn gives more confidence to the other player (with less skill) who now believes that he can win Thus, now it gets even harder for the better player to regain his confidence because he is playing against a now confident opponent.

This is why, at times, you see a highly ranked player lose to a lesser player in the early rounds of a tournament. The better player is often not particularly motivated, and in fact is oftentimes overconfident in his ability to beat this weaker opponent. So he doesn't prepare well physically and mentally and just thinks by showing up he will win. But this overconfidence (or false confidence) will usually lead to the higher ranked player being upset early and watching the rest of the tournament from the grandstands. I always felt that one of the truly great records of all time was the fact that over a 15 year period, Chris Evert reached at least the semi-finals in 44 of 45 Grand Slam tournaments. One might say that the women's draws were not as deep and tough as they are today and you would probably be right. But that doesn't take away from the unbelievable consistency of Chris Evert, which in part, has to be attributed to her lack of false confidence. She took all players seriously and prepared well for all her matches, whether early or late rounds. This exemplary record (and how it was achieved) should serve as a model for all tennis players to follow.

Assessing Confidence

Now that we know there is an optimal level of confidence and that we can be overconfident or lack confidence, it would be important to identify those areas within our tennis game. Table 5.2 is provided to help you locate your strengths and weaknesses in terms of confidence. To score your overall confidence, add up the percentages in each of the three columns and then divide each by 20. The higher your score on the "Confident Just Right" column, the more likely you are to be at your optimal level of confidence during a match. High scores on "Not Confident Enough" or "Confident Too Much" present some potential problem areas. To get a better sense of your specific strengths and weaknesses, look carefully at each item. You will notice that some of these are more related to your physical skills (e.g., confidence in your serve and volley) whereas others are concerned with your mental skills (e.g., confidence to make critical decisions in a match). This assessment should help target some specific areas of improvement in terms of your confidence.

Building Confidence

Now that we know our areas of strength as well as areas of improvement, we can turn to ways to enhance our feelings of confidence. Unfortunately, many tennis players make the mistake of thinking that there is not really anything they can do to improve their confidence.

Remember that one of the main themes of this book is that mental skills are indeed skills; therefore they can be learned, but need to be practiced. You will also note that several of these confidence-building techniques relate directly to the sources of confidence we discussed earlier.

Establish an Agreement With Yourself

Building and maintaining your confidence is both an important and challenging task. It is not easy to build self-confidence in tennis since it is an intricate, highly skillful, exacting, and at times exasperating sport. For example, many more points (even at the professional level) are won due to unforced errors as opposed to winners which is one reason why tennis can undermine one's confidence pretty quickly. This is especially the case on slower surfaces such as clay. As a top collegiate player recently said to me regarding errors on clay,

> *If you hit out and miss, then you chastise yourself for not playing more consistently and conservatively, just keeping the ball in play. But if you hit conservatively, and your opponent hits a winner or forcing shot, then you again berate yourself, this time for not going for your shots. You can't win either way.*

To prevent a loss of confidence and keep your focus positive and upbeat, I recommend that you make a personal agreement with yourself. This agreement should include the following elements as described below.

- *Do not doubt yourself.* We will discuss self-doubts in more detail in Chapter 7 as well as how to effectively deal with other negative thoughts. But you should make a commitment to staying confident and not getting down on yourself.
- *Give your best.* You will give undivided attention to your tennis and play each point in both practice and competition with a high level of concentration and effort.
- *You are not perfect.* You will agree that you are not perfect and that trying to be perfect is not realistic or helpful to you or your tennis. This is why so many players get so mad at themselves and upset when they miss shots. Many tennis players think they never should miss an easy shot (unforced error) but this is part of the game. Since nobody is perfect, this type of thinking just sets you up for failure. So if you recognize that you can learn from your mistakes and use them as a way to improve (as opposed to just putting yourself down) then this will go a long way toward enhancing your improvement.
- *Maintain your worth as a person.* Sometimes tennis players equate their performance on the court with their worth as a person. However, you will always maintain your worth as a person, regardless of how you might be playing on the court.
- *View events as positive challenges.* You will view pressure situations and quality opponents as positive challenges that make tennis fun and worthwhile. These situations will challenge you to do your best.

- *Expect to give maximum effort all the time.* You will anticipate giving full effort every time you play and thus expect to play well both in practice and competition. Effort is under your control, and simply expect to give it every time out on the court.

Performance Accomplishments

It gives you a lot of confidence beating a player three straight times. I knew if I do the things I do well, I should win.

Lindsay Davenport after beating Jelena Dokic
in the 2001 WTA Tour Championships

The above quote highlights the importance of past accomplishments as a source of confidence and as a way to build confidence. In fact, research and practice have clearly shown that the most powerful source of self-confidence is performance accomplishments. As noted earlier, these accomplishments fall into the categories of mastering skills and comparing your skills to others. But at its most basic level, performance accomplishments refer to performing well in the past (either mastering skills or winning competitions), which increases your confidence that you will be successful in the future. These could be mental skills such as effectively coping with pressure, pre-match preparation, or physical skills like hitting backhand passing shots or serving a high percentage.

Although it may sound easy, it is not always easy to build confidence this way. It is sometimes difficult to feel confident if you're not winning or playing well. Conversely, if you're not confident, you're probably not going to play well or win. Thus, it's kind of a "Catch-22." How do you build confidence if you're not successful, and how are you going to be successful if you're not confident? This dilemma is captured by the comments of a top touring professional who was in the middle of a hot streak, *I'm winning now because I'm confident, but the reason I'm confident is because I'm winning.*

Research in sport psychology, however, has revealed that for the most part, performance accomplishments enhance confidence and then confidence, in turn, enhances performance. So, how do we increase performance accomplishments? Of course, one way to enhance confidence through performance accomplishments is through setting up practices to hit certain shots or to practice certain mental abilities (or both). You will certainly feel more confidence in matches if you can execute different skills in practice on a consistent level. For example, let's say you are lacking confidence in your second serve, especially at critical points in matches. So you might decide to work exclusively on your second serve for 15 extra minutes each practice emphasizing depth, spin, and placement (you might set some specific goals using the principles from Chapter 4). In any case, just working on second serves is no replacement for having to hit serves at critical points in a match, like late in the third set. So you would need to set up pressure situations like hitting a second serve

Table 5.2	Tennis Confidence Inventory

This inventory will help you to evaluate your confidence about various characteristics of yourself that are important to being successful in tennis. As you know, tennis players can have too little confidence, too much confidence, or just about the right amount of confidence. Read each question and carefully think about your confidence with regard to each item as you competed over the past year. For each item, indicate, the percent of time you have too little, too much, or just the right amount of confidence. Below is an example to give you some idea about how to complete this inventory correctly.

	Not Confident Enough	Confidence Just Right	Too Much Confidence
How confident are you that you will get 60% of your first serves in?	40%	50%	10% = 100%

The total percent for all three answers should always be 100%. You may distribute this 100% in any way you think is appropriate. You may assign all 100% to one category, split it between two categories, or, as in the example, divide it among three categories. Remember, you are to indicate the percent of time when you compete in tennis, that you have too little, just about the right amount, or too much confidence.

With respect to your ability…	Not Confident Enough	Confidence Just Right	Too Much Confidence
1. To win from the baseline	_____%	_____%	_____%
2. To perform under pressure	_____%	_____%	_____%
3. To concentrate throughout a match	_____%	_____%	_____%
4. To serve and volley	_____%	_____%	_____%
5. To return serve successfully	_____%	_____%	_____%
6. To control your emotions in a match	_____%	_____%	_____%
7. To successfully approach the net	_____%	_____%	_____%
8. To hit backhand passing shots	_____%	_____%	_____%
9. To anticipate your opponent's shots	_____%	_____%	_____%
10. To come from behind and win	_____%	_____%	_____%

Table 5.2	Tennis Confidence Inventory cont.			
11. To hit backhand passing shots	_____%	_____%	_____%
12. To execute successful strategy	_____%	_____%	_____%
13. To improve your game	_____%	_____%	_____%
14. To put forth the effort to succeed	_____%	_____%	_____%
15. To consistently serve well	_____%	_____%	_____%
16. To hit forehand passing shots	_____%	_____%	_____%
17. To hit winners on your overhead	_____%	_____%	_____%
18. To outthink your opponent	_____%	_____%	_____%
19. To keep unforced errors low	_____%	_____%	_____%
20. To consistently hit with depth	_____%	_____%	_____%
Total	_____%	_____%	_____%
Total/20	_____%	_____%	_____%

at 4-5, 30-30, or 5-5, 30-40 so you could feel pressure like in a match. The more success you have in hitting your second serve under a variety of conditions, the more confidence you will have to hit it at critical points in a match.

Unfortunately, many players tend to focus on their strengths in practice, as opposed to working on their weaknesses. Of course if your volleys are not very good and you're not feeling confident up at net, you tend to stay away from net in practice. But the only way you are going to build confidence in your net game is to practice it again and again. Then you have to feel confident enough to use it in a match (which is easier said than done). I remember watching Steffi Graf over the years and she almost exclusively relied on her slice when hitting her backhand (which was a very underrated shot in my opinion). But if you saw her practice, she hit a wonderful topspin backhand that would be especially effective in hitting passing shots. Yet, she rarely used a topspin backhand in a match because she had so much confidence in her slice and never built up a strong sense of confidence in her topspin backhand (of course this didn't hurt her performance too much). But the point is that you have to take your performance accomplishments from the practice courts to matches in order to really build confidence in particular shots. In fact, research (Gould, Hodge, Peterson & Giannini, 1989; Weinberg & Jackson, 1990) has shown that coaches rely predominantly on "drilling and instruction" in order to build confidence. In essence, learning and performing shots and skills in practice, helps to build confidence to be transferred to actual matches.

Think Confidently

One of the key aspects of building and maintaining confidence is to think in a confident manner while on the court. In essence, this is making sure that you stay positive and say positive things to yourself, regardless of the situation, or how you happen to be performing on a given day or during a certain match. It is easy to be positive when everything is going well, but your confidence and positive thoughts will be tested when you have to deal with adversity and are not playing well. We will discuss the idea of thinking positively in more detail in Chapter 9, when we focus on "self-talk," but a few points are instructive at this point.

If you think confidently, your body is more likely to react in a confident manner. In fact, I would go so far as to say that keeping a positive attitude is essential if you want to be a successful tennis player. As one touring professional has said, *if I think I can win, then I'm awfully tough to beat.* The reason for this is that positive self-talk not only can provide specific performance cues, but it also can keep motivation and energy high, Although sometimes difficult to do, positive self-talk results in a more enjoyable and successful experience on the tennis court. So this means trying to eliminate all negative thoughts such as "You are an idiot", "How can you hit such a stupid shot," "you just can't beat this guy," and "you suck," and replacing these with more positive comments such as "just keep calm and focused," "hang in there, this match isn't over," or "just watch the ball." These positive thoughts should be instructive or help keep motivation up, especially during difficult times. As noted above, we will discuss self-talk in detail more in Chapter 9.

Act Confidently

One of the basic tenets of this book is that thoughts, feelings, emotions, and behaviors are interrelated and affect one another. Therefore, the more you behave in a confident manner, the more likely you are to feel and think confidently. This is especially important when things aren't going your way and your confidence level is low, as your opponent typically picks up on this and begins to gain confidence.

No matter how you are feeling or how the match is going, you should always display a confident image on the court. Both Serena and Venus Williams act confidently on the court (although they appear to be genuinely confident individuals) at all times which can really get into the head of an opponent. Along these lines, years ago, Chris Evert and Bjorn Borg never let an opponent know when they were not feeling confident (which probably was not often). Their expressions, movements, and mannerisms remained constant regardless of whether they were winning 5-1 or losing 5-1. The message that the opponents received was that these players had everything under their control and were not worried about losing (and certainly they were not going to stop trying on all points). Therefore, opponents never picked up any signals that these players had lost their confidence or desire, and couldn't use this information to infuse their own confidence.

Unfortunately, many players give themselves away due to their body language and movements, which indicate that they are lacking in confidence. Yelling at yourself, and throwing the racquet in disgust are just a couple of examples of how not acting confidently can not only fuel your opponent's emotions, but also undermine your own confidence. In fact, in one study, hundreds of matches (at least parts of matches) were videotaped and results revealed that observers could tell most of the time who was winning and losing, by simply watching how players moved and walked between points. Therefore, how players behave and carry themselves really provides important cues as to how they are actually performing on the court.

So acting confidently, can not only keep your opponent from feeding off your negativity, but it can also keep your own spirits up, even during difficult times in a match. If you walk around with slumped shoulders, dragged racquet, head down, and a painful facial expression, you communicate to your opponent that you are down, and this also works to pull you further down. Therefore, try to keep your shoulders back, head up, racquet head high, and facial muscles loose. This will send a signal to your opponent that you are confident and still fighting for the match. In turn, this will help your own level of confidence and keep you focused and into the match.

Visualize Positive Outcomes

One excellent way to improve your confidence is through visualizing success (we will discuss imagery in depth in Chapter 8). One of the prime benefits of using imagery is that you can see yourself doing things on the court that maybe you had difficulty in accomplishing in the past. For example, you might have trouble consistently executing a slice backhand deep in to the court or hitting a flat serve down the middle of the court. Along these lines, certain situations might also cause you difficulty such as returning a hard serve or serving out a match. Similarly, you might have been defeated several times in a row by a particular player and feel discouraged when having to play this person. But one of the neat things about imagery is that you can visualize being successful against this opponent and carrying out your game plan flawlessly. Or you can see yourself executing the slice backhand and serve that has given you trouble in the past as well as reacting positively (keeping calm and staying with your game plan) to serving out a match. Whatever the scenario, imagery can help you create successful situations, which brings with it a sense of confidence that you can execute these skills or play well against a specific opponent.

Increase Physical Fitness Levels

In recent years, being in top physical condition has become more and more a part of being successful in tennis at the top levels (as well as lower levels). Years ago, like in many sports, physical fitness and conditioning were not stressed: rather it was purely the development of the skills related to that sport. But this changed, especially with the physical training regimens (and subsequent success) of players like Martina Navratilova and Ivan Lendl and more recently, Jim Courier, Andre Agassi, and Lindsay Davenport. So no longer was preparation for tennis just on the court hitting shots. Rather, lifting weights, running, proper nutrition, rest, and other conditioning exercises, have become important if a player is to get into top physical shape. It certainly is a source of confidence when you feel that you are in top shape and can stay out on the court all day if necessary.

This has especially been the case for Andre Agassi and his resurgence at a relatively late age for a professional tennis player (around 30 year old). He has repeatedly said that being in the best shape of his life gives him confidence on the tennis court since he feels that he can outlast anyone in a long match. This is not just talk, as anyone who has watched Agassi play, has realized that he no longer goes for outright winners very often; rather he is content to move his opponents around from side to side with angles and "safe" shots, since he feels that the longer the point (and the match) goes on, the better chance he has of winning. This helped him win the French Open and become the only active player with wins at all four Grand Slams. His commitment to fitness has given him the confidence to play at the top of his game.

Establish a Clear Game Plan

Before playing the first point of a match, it is necessary to have in mind a game plan, which is a basic set of guidelines for your play. This does not mean that you have a strategy for every shot that you hit. Rather, a game plan requires that you have a general idea of what you want to accomplish and how you want to accomplish it. A solid game plan that a player believes in, can be an important part to building a player's confidence. In essence, a game plan gives your efforts structure and direction, without which you are hitting balls that have no specific purpose. Thus, it helps build confidence because you know what you're going to try to do. This will usually involve trying to break down an opponent's weakness and understanding what you need to do to win points. Even if you don't know your opponent, you should construct a game plan based on your own strengths and weaknesses

A game plan is kind of funny in that it must be taken seriously enough to commit your full mental energy to its execution, yet not seriously enough, that it is rigid and you cannot adjust it. Therefore, at the start of a match you need to commit to your game plan and its execution. However, you also have to monitor the progress of the match and see if your game plan is working satisfactorily. If you are losing and your initial game plan is not working, then you must seriously consider changing your game plan. The great champion Bill Tilden is credited with coining the old adage, *Always change a losing game; never change a winning game.* Of course this makes good sense but it isn't always easy to determine when your game is a losing one and thus you should change your plan. For example, what if you lose the first set 6-4 and the major part of your plan was to come to the net as often as possible against your opponent's weaker backhand. You were sometimes successful with this tactic and other times you were passed. So, should you change your game plan?

Most players tend to make the mistake of giving up on a game plan too early or changing it too drastically. Unfortunately, there are no hard and fast rules that apply to changing game plans. But in general, as soon as things start to go wrong, most players suspect their strategy is at fault and they get panicky and emotional. They quickly try something else and typically their alternative game plan is worse than their initial plan. But sometimes changing game plans is the right thing to do. If you do this, make sure the new game plan is within your capabilities. But often, capabilities are not evaluated accurately. For example, you might be capable of successfully serving and volleying only 30% of the time. So it might not be a good idea to change your baseline game to a serve and volley game, just because your game plan of slugging it out from the baseline is not working (you are generally pretty steady from the baseline except your opponent is out steadying you on this day). I like to define capabilities (in relation to game plans) as those that do not lead to a substantial increase in your error rate. In essence the serve and volley strategy mentioned above would not be within your capabilities, since your percentage of errors goes up drastically. But tennis is also a game played over some time and what is working early does not always work later. So if your game plan of breaking down your opponent's weaker backhand was not working in the first set, it may work in the second set when your opponent starts to feel a little pressure. But if you abandoned your game plan too early, then you might not really test your opponent's backhand under pressure. Thus, having a game plan that you are confident in, and will try to execute across a match (given clear evidence that it is not working), will help remove uncertainty, which should increase confidence (game plans are discussed in more detail in Chapter 10).

Staying Confident During Adverse Situations

One of the most discouraging times for a tennis player is when you are playing pretty well, but your opponent can't miss (maybe he is in the zone). Even though you might be doing all the right things and playing as well as you can, your opponent seems to have all the answers. At this point, your confidence can really take a beating if you don't handle the situation correctly. Many players just give up because they feel that they can't possibly beat this particular player on this given day. Or maybe you start going for low percentage shots (many times shots that are outside of your normal repertoire) since you feel this is the only way you can win a point.

A confident tennis player realizes that players sometimes go through hot streaks, but these players will usually cool off after several games or a set. It is rare that a player can go though an entire match with such a high level of shot making and consistency. The key is to maintain your confidence and keep the level of your game high so when your opponent falters, you are right there to take advantage of the situation. This is easier said than done, because it is difficult to retain your confidence and stay upbeat when you continue to lose points and games due to your opponent's high standard of play. Confident players, however, feel that if they keep the pressure on, their opponent will typically break sooner or later.

The key is not to let the level of your game fall, even though your opponent is on a hot streak. I remember the great Arthur Ashe saying that when his opponent is playing "out of his mind," he would try to raise the level of his game 10-15% (even if he was still losing points) so that he would be in a position to take over the match when his opponent eventually faltered a little.

The same can be said when you are going through a rough patch where you can't seem to keep the ball in play and maybe you have lost your rhythm on a particular shot or in your entire game. Again, it's easy to lose confidence and get down on yourself. But you have to remember that early performance is not a good or consistent predictor of later performance. So if you're not playing well early in a match, if you keep your confidence up, then you are more likely to play well later in the match. Many of the strategies noted in this chapter can be used to help keep your confidence high such as thinking confidently (i.e., positively) and acting confidently even if you don't feel particularly confident at that moment.

CHAPTER 6

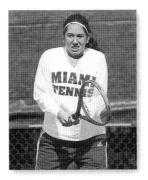

UNDERSTANDING AND MANAGING YOUR EMOTIONS

You know from playing tennis that emotions play an important role in how well you play as well as the final outcome of a match. As noted earlier, tennis is not merely about stroke production, mechanics and technique. Sport psychologists (as well as competitive tennis players) have long understood managing anxiety, arousal, and emotions are critical to performing at high levels. But what are some of the sources of a player's anxiety? How does a player find his or her optimal level of arousal? What techniques are there to lower and increase arousal? These are just some of the questions we will try to address in this chapter. But let's start with a few quotes that highlight the notion that emotions can act in either a positive or negative manner.

I like to fire up, to feel the adrenaline flowing; that's when I play my best.

Chris Evert

I thrive on emotions. They're reflected in my game with aggressive play; with going forward all the time…and with a heightened awareness of what's going on that I'd compare to an animal's instinct in hunting down its prey. The emotional energy allows me to raise the level of my play.

Jimmy Connors

Before a match I'm so high strung that by the warm-ups I'm completely wiped out, both mentally and physically. This leads to negative thinking, as I lose my focus, play recklessly, and then just cash in my chips.

Collegiate Tennis Player

Sometimes when I go out on the court to play an important match, I get so nervous that I actually have trouble breathing. I feel tension all over and when I try to run, my legs feel stiff and tight, making me slow around the court. I start pushing my shots with little or no follow-through. It seems that I lose my tennis instincts and I become controlled by a fear of failure.

Competitive Junior Tennis Player

The above quotes demonstrate the range of positive and negative outcomes that increases in anxiety and arousal can bring to one's tennis game. As we will note later in the chapter, the concept of individual differences in response to pressure situations is critical. Once again Jimmy Connors is "right on" with the following comments.

I liked to clench my fists and pump my arms on big points and big shots, but this type of behavior is not for everyone. It worked for me, but you shouldn't try to pattern your emotional responses after someone else's. What works for the person you're imitating may not work for you. And it's impossible to play at a feverish emotional peak for long; you would just use up too much energy in trying to keep you at that high level.

The latest research in sport psychology has supported these anecdotal claims that anxiety can sometimes be seen as facilitative as well as debilitative. But before we address the relationship between anxiety and performance, it is important to understand that anxiety comes in two different types—*somatic and cognitive*. Somatic anxiety refers to the physiological aspects of anxiety such as a racing heart, increased breathing rate, muscle tension, "butterflies" in the stomach, and feet feeling heavy. The cognitive aspect of anxiety refers to the worry component and is characterized by negative self-talk, fear of failure, and worrying about the consequences of your actions. Now that we know what anxiety is, let us discuss what research tells us regarding the sources of anxiety for tennis players.

Sources of Anxiety

In interviews with over a thousand athletes, results revealed that the number one thing preventing them from reaching their potential as an athlete was the failure to effectively cope with anxiety before and during competition. This result alone says a lot about the critical role that anxiety plays in athletic performance. Certainly, tennis is a game in which players have to regularly and consistently deal with pressurized situations. Research has clearly revealed that the ability to effectively cope with anxiety is certainly one of the characteristics of elite performers and this is seen in the tennis world as illustrated by the comments of a current top tour professional.

I can think of many, many players that nobody has ever heard of (world rankings in the hundreds) who can hit the ball as well and as hard as anyone on the tour but just can't get it together for matches. The reason that guys like Sampras, Agassi, Hewitt, and Kuerten are champions (or up and coming champions) is that they always play their best on big points in key matches and tournaments. Most players either get a little tentative on big points or choose high risk, low percentage shots. But these guys go for their shots, but at the same time play within their abilities.

As a tennis player or coach, you first have to recognize and understand what causes anxiety before you can begin to effectively cope with it. Table 6.1 provides a questionnaire to help assess the different specific sources of anxiety for yourself. Although there are many sources of anxiety, research has revealed the following three major sources of competitive anxiety.

Table 6.1	Sources of Anxiety

Instructions: The purpose of this exercise is to help you determine what stressful situations are occurring in your matches. Listed below are some reasons why tennis players worry and become anxious. Write the number that best represents how you generally feel during tennis matches (all statements begin with "I worry about"..). Look over your responses when you complete this worksheet and this should help determine your most anxiety-producing situations.

1 = almost always   to   7 = almost never

Anxiety Source	1	2	3	4	5	6	7
What my coach will think or say							
What my parents will think or say							
Making mistakes							
Losing							
Not playing well							
Not being able to concentrate							
How I feel before the match							
Losing my temper							
Playing in championship matches							
How well my opponent is playing							
How I look							
Feeling weak							
Line calls							

Fear of Failure

Fear of failure is the most prevalent reason given by tennis players for what makes them nervous and anxious. The immediate fear usually centers around losing a match, missing a shot, blowing a big opportunity on an important point, or just looking bad. But the real reason for fear of failure usually resides in threats to self-esteem and self-worth. So the real fear of failure is evidenced in statements such as, "What will other people think if I lose?" "I am only as good as how I play on the tennis court," "I'll never be able to face my friends if I lose this first round match," and "I don't want to disappoint my teammates, coach, and parents."

In essence, a tennis match becomes much more than just a competition between two players, as the consequences go beyond the realm of the tennis court. In reality, you think that somehow you are a better person, or will be more liked if you win, or conversely, that you are a lesser person or will not be as well-liked if you lose. This, of course, can place great pressure on a player, if your ego is so tied up in the outcome of a match. That is why it was good to hear Boris Becker's comments after losing a first round match at Wimbledon to a player who had not won a match all year up until that time. *All I lost was a tennis match. It was not a war and nobody got killed.* In short, Becker was saying that it wasn't the end of the world if he lost a tennis match (even if it was at Wimbledon where he was one of the best players in the history of tennis).

When you have a fear of failure, you usually will play not to lose instead of playing to win. This translates into playing very conservatively, not going for your shots, and hoping the opponent will make some unforced errors. Although this strategy might work occasionally at the lower levels of skill where your opponent is not capable of taking advantage of your tentative play, it is not effective as players become more skilled and will "make you pay" for your tentative shots. The idea of playing with a fear of failure is nicely summarized by Andre Agassi.

> What I've learned from others is that it can mess you up if you worry about every-body, worry about winning, hoping to be the next great American player. What peo-ple want to think is their business. I'm just going to play the way I want to play. I'm not going to be afraid to lose. If I start worrying about losing, I'll never win.

Feelings of Inadequacy

Typically speaking, feelings of inadequacy are concerned with feeling inadequately prepared either physically or mentally. Tennis players report such things as feeling inadequate about their physical conditioning, inability to maintain concentration, lack of desire to play, inability to control anxiety, and lack of rest. This state is especially characterized by the attitude of "something is wrong with me." In essence, tennis players report that they feel ill at ease due to their inability to properly prepare (both physically and mentally) for an upcoming competition. It is important that players feel adequately prepared about their training so that they can approach a match with confidence and low anxiety. This is noted by 12 time Grand Slam winner Roy Emerson.

> *Any time you walk on a tennis court in less than top physical shape you're giving your-self a convenient reason for losing. When I was playing on the circuit, I knew that there were players who had better strokes than I, but I had confidence in my body. I knew I had trained harder and prepared myself better than the other guy, and I knew that if it came down to a fifth set, he was more likely to wilt than was I.*
>
> *(Tarshis 1977, p. 170)*

Players such as Jim Courier, Steffi Graf, Amanda Coetzer, Michael Chang, Arantxa Sanchez Vicario, and more recently, Andre Agassi, have long been noted for their preparation. This preparation helped build their confidence and keep their anxiety levels low while also helping them get the most out of their ability.

Loss of Control

Another consistent factor relating to tennis players' anxiety is their feeling of control. When players feel out of control, their anxiety levels tend to rise and they can easily become frustrated, annoyed, and impatient. For example, one area where many players feel a loss of control is in line calls. I have heard players often attribute a loss to a bad line call (or series of bad calls) as this is a convenient excuse for losing. Of course there is nothing much you can do about line calls, but if you fixate on them, then this will take your focus out of the game, and at the same time increase your anxiety. Players with more self-control realize that matches rarely are won or lost on a line call, and you just have to take the good with the bad.

Other situations that are out of your control on the tennis court include, wind, sun, temperature, spectators, type of playing surface (e.g., grass, clay, hard court), and conduct of your opponent. These also can produce feelings of anxiety as most players don't like to play when it's windy, the sun is right in their eyes, and the court is not to their liking. For example, even though most players do not like wind, some players will in fact be beat before they ever step out on the court saying , "I can't play in the wind." But there are things you can do when playing in the wind that are under your control such as hitting harder against the wind and putting more topspin on the ball to keep it in with the wind. The key point is that loss of control can promote anxiety so you need to stay in control when certain events are out of your control. When practicing mental skills, it is instructive to know what is under your control and what is not since you want to focus on things that are in your control. This sometimes gets muddied during competition, so Table 6.2 provides some examples of things in and out of your control. Feel free to add to this list and make sure you focus on things within your control.

| Table 6.2 | Factors You Can and Cannot Control |

It's important to focus on changing only those things that are in your control and not waste emotional energy on things out of your control (which can sometimes be a source of stress). So I'll provide a partial list (and you can add to the list) of factors that you can and cannot control.

Can Control	Cannot Control
Your mental state	The weather
How you feel	Your parent's (coach's) actions
Your response to situations	Your opponent's actions
Your intensity level	A string breaking
Your thoughts	The court surface
How you act	Opponent's line calls
Your confidence	Your tournament draw

Excess Anxiety—Physical Effects

Now that you understand some of the prime causes of anxiety, it would be instructive to consider how excess anxiety can affect you both physically and mentally. This requires a brief understanding of the *flight-or-fight* response, which occurs as the body prepares itself for a threatening situation. In essence, it gives you the ability to react quickly to danger. The problem occurs when this system is activated, for example, in preparing or playing a big tennis match. The body can prepare for this situation with excess levels of adrenaline, which makes it difficult to perform the fine motor skills with the precision that is required in tennis. Below are a couple of specific physical problems caused by excess anxiety.

Muscle Tension

Probably the most debilitating and typical response to excess anxiety is that muscles tense beyond appropriate levels. To hit a tennis ball properly requires that some muscles need to be tense while others should be relaxed. For example, in hitting with topspin, you need to have a loose wrist to come over the ball. But if your forearm and wrist muscles are too tight, this will prevent you from rotating over the ball. Players tend to "tighten up" at critical points in a match because they feel too much tension and pressure. We will discuss how to cope with this excess tension a little later in the chapter.

Reduced Flexibility

A second problem with excess anxiety is that it reduces flexibility, which is also usually caused by excess muscle tension. For example, when serving, you have to drop the racquet head to the "scratch your back" position, which allows for greater velocity and wrist snap. But when you are feeling too tight due to excess muscle tension, your back swing is reduced, resulting in less velocity and usually less control. Unfortunately, many tennis players contract all of their muscles when trying to hit a big serve (I once was one of these players) which usually results in not only less power, but also less accuracy. Along with reduced flexibility comes an increased probability of injury since muscles can't go through the entire range of motion.

Fatigue

A third problem with excess anxiety is that it produces fatigue in the muscles involved. Contracting a muscle for a prolonged period of time can produce fatigue, which typically will result in poorer performance as the match progresses. This is one reason why you see professional players rolling their heads around in order to reduce tension and fatigue in the neck and shoulder area.

Excess Anxiety-Mental Effects

Besides causing some physical problems, excess anxiety can also negatively affect you from a mental point of view. These psychological detrimental effects include impaired concentration, poor decision-making, and reduced confidence.

Reduced Concentration

Research has clearly revealed that excess anxiety can distract you from focusing on the task at hand. When you are anxious, you are likely to focus on worries rather than on the point being played. For example, if you're playing an important match and you are overly concerned with the outcome, then you might be thinking about winning and losing, rather than simply playing the upcoming point. In addition, you might be worried about what your parents might think, how this match might affect your rankings, or what people might think of you if you lose? In any case, your concentration is focused on distracting and meaningless thoughts as they have nothing to do with you winning the next point and game. We will discuss the relationship between anxiety and attention in Chapter 7.

Impaired Decision-Making

Another area in which excess anxiety can cause problems is with decision-making. Tennis is a game of decisions and playing the percentages. I have often seen players with better strokes and physical ability lose to lesser players because they let anxiety impact their decision-making and shot selection. When matches get tight and pressure starts to mount, players have a tendency to forget their game plan and start to choose ill-advised (i.e., low percentage) shots. For example, you might have a game plan to approach net whenever possible against an opponent's weaker backhand. But serving at 5-4 for the set you get passed on an approach. So you get anxious and decide not to approach the net anymore, which is totally opposite to your well thought-out game plan. To discard your game plan due to one shot is usually a bad decision.

However, becoming anxious may not only affect your choice of shot, but also how to hit a particular shot. This sometimes leads to going for too much because the longer a point goes on, the more anxiety builds up. Thus, the player chooses a low-percentage shot in order to end the point, one way or another. But sometimes the opposite occurs, as a player may start to "push" the ball, in order to avoid making a mistake (I see this often in junior matches where there is 30 feet of net clearance on each shot). But against a better player, this is a poor decision as he or she will eventually take the offensive and often force the "pusher" into a mistake. In either case, anxiety is the culprit that produced a strategy inconsistent with maximizing your chance of being successful and playing up to your potential.

Reduced Confidence

Research has revealed that there is an inverse relationship between anxiety and confidence. In other words, as anxiety gets higher, confidence becomes lower. We know from Chapter 5 that confidence is critical for optimal performance. However, when you are feeling very anxious, it is highly difficult, if not impossible, to feel confident in your abilities. I have detailed many of the negative side-effects of not being confident, which usually means not going for your shots, getting down on yourself (especially when behind), not trying hard at all times, and a lack of belief in your abilities.

Arousal-Performance Relationship

Now that we know what causes anxiety and how it might impact performance, let's take a closer look at the relationship between arousal and performance. Many theories have been developed to help explain the arousal-performance relationship but one constant if that most theories indicate that there is an optimal level of arousal, which is related to a player's best performance. We will take a look at one such approach, which considers players' individual differences in their reaction to arousal levels.

Zones of Optimal Functioning

Some excellent research by Yuri Hanin (1997- formerly of the Soviet Union), as well as others, has found that different athletes have different optimal levels of arousal. In essence, some people seem to perform best at low levels of arousal, others are at their best at moderate levels, whereas others perform best at high levels of arousal (see Figure 6.1). Everyone has a particular optimal level, but that level varies across individuals. That is why it is important not to compare yourself to other players, because all tennis players function differently. For example, Pete Sampras generally does not display a lot of emotion, whereas Lleyton Hewitt is constantly slapping his leg and verbally exhorting himself to increase his arousal. On the women's side, Lindsay Davenport is typically non-emotional, whereas the Williams sisters (Venus and Serena) seem to help generate and feed off high arousal levels. These differences are usually related to our personality styles and that is why it is best to choose the style best suited for you, rather than trying to copy the style of a particular player (which may be at odds with your comfort zone).

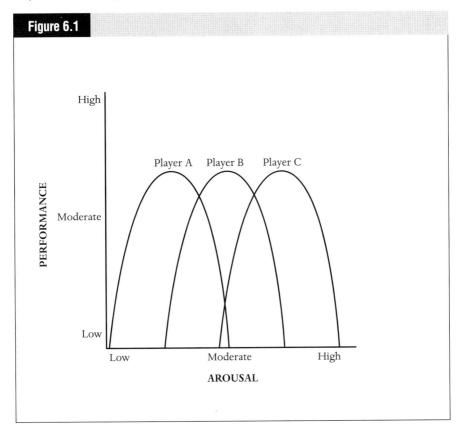

Figure 6.1

Finding Your Optimal Arousal Level

Now that you know that each player has a different optimal arousal level, the trick is to find that special level. This can be done on a more scientific level or simply by "feel" as many athletes do. But no matter how you do it (and it isn't always an easy thing to do), your goal should be to consistently reach your optimal level of arousal for each match and tournament.

Thus, to find your optimal arousal level, you must determine what level you are at when you are performing at your best. One way to accomplish this is to complete the inventory provided in Table 6.3 which measures both your cognitive and somatic anxiety intensity level from 1 -11, and also asks whether you perceive this anxiety as facilitative or debilitative to performance. In recent years, Jones and his colleagues (Jones & Swain, 1995; Jones, Swain, & Hardy, 1993) have provided empirical support to the notion that anxiety levels can be seen as either helping or hindering sport performance. Before, high levels of anxiety were always seen as hurting performance but now we know it's not the actual levels themselves that count as much as what you do with them. In essence, it's how you view anxiety and how you cope with it that really are the key determinants of performance.

So what you should do is complete the form provided in Table 6.3 either before several matches or after several matches using the technique of retrospection. In this procedure, you

Table 6.3	Assessment of Cognitive and Somatic Anxiety

Please complete this scale either right before a competition (or right after thinking back to how you felt right before the competition in a retrospective manner). Choose the response that most aptly reflects how you are thinking and feeling right now. There are no right and wrong answers—this is for your own benefit.

For the intensity scale use   1 = not at all to 11 = very much so
For the direction scale use   1 = very facilitative to 11 = very debilitative

	Intensity	Direction
Somatic (Physical) Responses		
1. I feel anxious	_____	_____
2. I feel tension in my muscles	_____	_____
3. My body feels jittery	_____	_____
4. I am breathing quickly	_____	_____
5. My heart is racing	_____	_____
TOTAL	_____	_____
Cognitive (Thinking) Responses		
6. I have doubts about this performance	_____	_____
7. I am concerned about how I am going to do	_____	_____
8. I am worried about choking	_____	_____
9. I am concerned that I won't be able to focus	_____	_____
10. I am worried that I will lose	_____	_____
TOTAL	_____	_____

would think back to how you felt before the match and complete the inventory accordingly. You would then assess your performance on the tennis court either subjectively or objectively. If it is done objectively, then you would need to have someone recording things such as winners, unforced errors, first and second serve percentage, and service return points won (first and second serves). If you do it subjectively, then you (or possibly a coach) could rate yourself in relation to how you normally play from say "1" (much worse than usual) to "11" (much better than usual). You can use any scoring system you want—the main point is to get objective and subjective (if possible) evaluations of your performance on the tennis court.

Matching Best Performance With Anxiety Levels

Then you need to match up your best performances with your particular anxiety levels to create a zone of optimal functioning. For example, if you performed best at an intensity level of 35 for somatic anxiety (using the 1-11 scale provided) you could create a zone of between 32 and 38 (plus or minus 3 points). You would do the same thing for cognitive anxiety, as this would put you at your optimal level of arousal for peak performance. For example, if you knew that you performed best (after repeated assessments) when your somatic anxiety was 35 and your cognitive anxiety was 28 (given that you viewed these levels as facilitative to performance—which you probably would, because you performed best at these intensity levels), then you would attempt to regulate your anxiety levels to put yourself as close to these levels of anxiety as possible. (I will provide some techniques to control your anxiety levels later in this chapter). In any case you would try to create a zone of optimal functioning so that you are at your optimal level of somatic and cognitive anxiety. Once you find out about your optimal zone and understand how to get yourself there, then you will maximize your chances of performing up to your potential.

Reducing Anxiety

After completing several of these anxiety scales and assessing your performance, you should know what your optimal level of arousal should be to perform at your best. For most tennis players, the problem is that they are too anxious and need to relax more on the court. We have discussed the many different negative side effects of excess anxiety both physically and mentally. For example, excess anxiety can produce inappropriate and increased muscle tension, which can lead to performance decreases. Fortunately, most top tennis players are quite skillful at detecting very subtle increases in muscular tension, and they can make the necessary adjustments.

However, many recreational tennis players tend to tense up all their muscles when they get too anxious. For instance, when trying to hit with more power, it is best to relax the major muscle groups that work against the muscles required to perform a particular movement. But many players have difficulty doing this and just try to hit harder, contracting all their muscles. How many times have you tried to hit that big serve of yours, only to find that you don't really hit it that hard and you lose accuracy in the process? This is because trying harder does no always produce better performance. In fact, research has shown that athletes asked to give 90% effort will actually perform better than when given instructions to give 100% or even 110% effort. The problem is that when athletes are told to give 100%, they simply contract their muscles (this is the natural thing to do) and expect that this will produce the most effort and the best performance. However, skilled performance, requires an intricate interplay between having some muscles relaxed while other are contracting. Simply trying to relax won't work. We have to learn how to relax. This will be the focus of the next section in which I will present some established techniques for lowering anxiety levels.

Breath Control

One of the easiest yet most effective ways to control anxiety and tension is through proper breathing. Of course, most of us take breathing for granted because we do it every minute of every day. But the pressure of a tennis match can change the way you normally breathe making your breathing short, shallow, and irregular, instead of smooth, deep, and rhythmical. One common mistake made by tennis players when playing under pressure is failing to coordinate their breathing with their stroke production. Research has indicated that breathing in and holding your breath increases muscle tension, whereas breathing out decreases muscle tension. Some top players like Monica Seles are known as "grunters" because they appear to grunt after every shot. But what this really does is ensure that she breathes out (exhales) whenever she hits the ball. Unfortunately, many tennis players actually hold their breath while stroking the ball, which simply adds to the muscle tension and interferes with smooth stroke production.

Many tennis players take breaths that are too shallow—their chests expands, their shoulders rise, and their gut remains sucked in. Although this may look good, it is not effective breathing. Rather, '"belly breathing" where you breathe deeply and slowly while drawing the air in all the way down to your abdomen, is a more effective way to breathe. Let's briefly look at what you need to do to practice breath control.

Practicing Breath Control

To practice breath control, you should focus on doing the following.

1. Inhale deeply and slowly through your nose and as you do, notice how your body seems to lift up. Breathe from your stomach and diaphragm and then let the air taken in fill and expand the central and upper chest. Your stomach should be pushed fully outward, as the breath is taken in. This inhalation phase should last approximately four to five seconds.

2. Exhale slowly through your mouth in a very relaxed manner. You should feel the muscles in your arms and shoulders relax. As you breathe out and relax, you should begin to feel centered and anchored to the ground. The entire exhalation process

should last 8-10 seconds. It is important that the exhalation be done slowly, but at a steady rate, with approximately a 1:2 ratio of inhalation to exhalation. So if your inhalation is 3 seconds then the exhalation phase should be about 6 seconds.

Applying Breath Control

Although breath control can be practiced outside the court, it can also be employed on the court, during your strokes, between points, and during changeovers. One way to use breath control during play is to help you get into the rhythm of stroking. One scenario is to breathe out in relation to two cues: (a) when the ball bounces, and (b) when you make contact. Start to exhale when the ball bounces and don't inhale until after you make contact. To help learn this process, you might try to say the words "can't...miss" as cues once the ball bounces (or anything else that works for you). In essence, it's one long exhalation. This exhalation helps to focus all your energies on hitting the ball. You don't want to start your exhalation when you hit the ball (as some players do) because this will not allow you to hit with full energy as you release tension from when the ball hits the court.

You can help maintain your composure and control your anxiety during points by using breath control. Focusing on your breathing means you are not focusing on irrelevant cues such as the spectators or an opponent's antics. Many players like to use breathing as a way to calm themselves just prior to serving. This helps relax the shoulder and neck muscles, slow things down a bit (especially after a tough point), and keeps you focused on the next point. Finally, breathing can be used during changeover when you have 60-90 seconds to "gather yourself" and get ready for the next game. At this time, proper breathing can help focus and energize you while taking a brief mental break from the match.

Progressive Relaxation (Muscle Relaxation)

When it comes to achieving relaxation, probably the "gold standard" is known as Progressive Relaxation (PR) originally developed by Edmund Jacobson (1938). It is termed Progressive Relaxation because you progress from one muscle group to another until the major muscle groups are covered. The major tenets of PR include the following:

- Tension and relaxation are mutually exclusive. A muscle is either tense or relaxed. It cannot be sort of tense or sort of relaxed.
- Relaxation of the body through decreased muscular tension (somatic anxiety) will also decrease mental tension (cognitive anxiety).
- It is possible to learn the difference between a relaxed and tense muscle. These differences are sometimes subtle, but can be learned with practice.
- Progressive relaxation is accomplished by systematically relaxing and contracting the major muscle groups in the body.

General Instructions

You can purchase any of a number of audio tapes, that will help take you through PR, step-by-step. But here are some general points you should follow in practicing this technique.

- The basic idea is that you learn the difference between a tense and relaxed muscle (You should start in a relaxed, distraction-free environment such as sitting in an easy chair at home where there are no competing noises or sounds).
- To accomplish this, induce as much tension in a particular muscle (or muscle group) and hold that tension and try to feel it.
- Then relax that muscle as completely as possible and try to understand the difference between what a tense and relaxed muscle feel like.
- Both the tension and relaxation phases should take about 5-7 seconds each. Repeat this twice for each muscle group before moving on to the next muscle group.
- As you become more skilled, you will be able to identify tension in specific muscles and then be able to relax that muscle.
- The first few sessions might take up to 30 minutes but after that you should be able to start to relax in about 5 to 10 minutes.
- The final goal is cue-controlled relaxation where you will be able to relax based on a cue word you have learned such as "relax." This is what you would try to do on-court when feeling anxious.

Mental Relaxation (Relaxation Response)

Progressive Relaxation works from the physical to the mental. However, another way to accomplish relaxation is to first relax the mind, and then relax the body. This is the goal of the Relaxation Response developed by Herbert Benson (Benson & Proctor, 1984), a physician at the Harvard Medical School. The state of mind produced by this technique is characterized by keen awareness, effortlessness, relaxation, spontaneity, and focused attention. What is particularly interesting about this technique is that it produces many of the same elements tennis players use to describe their top performances (see Chapter 2). The technique should take about 20-30 minutes and the key elements are described below.

Specific Instructions

One of the nice things about this technique is that it is very simple and straightforward. It involves only four simple elements. These include the following:

- *Quiet Environment.* A quiet place is necessary where external stimulation and distractions are at a minimum.
- *Comfortable Position.* Assume a position that is comfortable for you and that you can maintain throughout the time required for this technique. There is no set position.
- *Mental Device.* This is the critical element in the Relaxation Response. It involves focusing on a single thought or word and repeating it over and over. Be sure to

select a word that has no particular meaning to you and does not stimulate your thoughts. Some people have successfully used words such as easy, calm, or relax, repeating their particular word in conjunction with breathing out (exhaling).

- *Passive Attitude.* This involves allowing thoughts to enter your mind, but to move through them in a passive manner, making no attempt to attend to them. If something comes into your mind, let it go and refocus your attention on your word.

By practicing this technique, you will likely find how difficult it is to control your mind and focus your attention on either one thought or object. But isn't the goal of concentrating during a point to stay focused on the ball and not let your mind wander? Furthermore, between points you must maintain your concentration, not letting irrelevant thoughts enter your mind (and if they do, get rid of them as soon as possible). Thus, the Relaxation Response can help you not only relax, but also to maintain concentration throughout a match.

On-Court-Relaxation Tips

Besides the techniques noted above, there are other things you can do to reduce anxiety on the court. Players I have worked with have often told me that just a simple reminder or cue can often have a profound impact on the quality of their play. So let's look at some of these tips.

16 Second Cure

One scientifically developed and practical method to regain control of your anxiety and other emotions between points is to employ the16 Second Cure developed by well-known sport psychologist Jim Loehr. The 16 Second Cure was designed specifically to help players structure their time between points or games to help them be better prepared for the next point. However, you might modify it slightly to fit your individual needs, personality and ability. It is comprised of four stages:

(a) *Positive Physical Response*—Following a lost point, make a quick decisive move away from the mistake as if to say with your body "no problem." Immediately transfer your racquet to your non-dominant hand with your head tilted up and walk back to your position with your shoulders back, head up, and eyes forward and down, projecting a strong, confident image.

(b) *Relaxation Response*—Once behind the baseline keep your feet moving. Your eyes should be looking at the strings of your racquet or at the ground. Shake out your arms if necessary to release tension. Always walk several feet behind the baseline before starting the next point. The more stressful the point, the more time you should take in this stage.

(c) *Preparation Response*—Move toward your serve or service return position. Project the strongest, most confident image possible. Now is when you should plan what you're going to do with the upcoming point. Know how you will play it.

(d) *Automatic Ritual Response*—If you're serving, bounce the ball at least two times and pause after the last bounce to gather yourself before starting the service motion. This will guard against hurrying when under pressure. If you're returning, fix your eyes on the ball on the other side. Maintain movement by jumping up and down or swaying back and forth. Some players like to spin their racquet in their hand or blow on their hands. The goal is to be completely prepared for the next point.

Use Cue Words

One of the best ways to relax in pressure situations is to use cue words that help you to remember to relax. Such words as *easy, calm,* and *relax* (similar to the mental device words suggested earlier) remind you to keep your muscles relaxed and your mind clear and focused. More on the use of cue words (especially in relation to self-talk) will be presented in Chapter 9.

Slow Down Between Points

Many players react to feeling pressure (and maybe being a little mad and frustrated) by starting to play too fast. This is easy to understand because anxiety and pressure are usually not desirable to a player, and one easy way to cope with this pressure is to hurry up and get off the court. When players play too fast they typically lose concentration and make bad decisions (go for too much—or in some cases just try to push the ball back instead of hitting a normal shot). When this rushing starts while serving, I typically tell the players I work with, to slow down by walking to the ball farthest away from them, and using that ball to serve with. This, combined with a consistent pre-service routine (see Chapter 8) will usually be enough to slow players down. When returning serve, you can pick up any balls on your side and take some deep breaths described earlier. Remember, the server can't serve until you're ready. That doesn't mean you should stall, but you should take your time and slow down, especially when things are not going well and you feel the match is slipping away from you.

Smile When You Feel Tension Coming On

Oftentimes, players take tennis too seriously, and feel the "weight of the world" on their shoulders. But tennis is just a game (we have to keep reminding ourselves of this point) and we need to remember to keep it in its proper perspective. One simple way to do this is to smile when you feel you are becoming tense and uptight. It is difficult to be mad and upset at the same time you are smiling. One top junior player I worked with used to falter under pressure, but she felt smiling was a little funny and beneath her. But in a match she found herself quickly down 3-0 and feeling lots of pressure (since she was expected to win this match). So she remembered what we had spoken about regarding smiling, and she said she simply put a big smile on her face. This evidently helped reduce the tension and loosened her up. She went on to win 5 games in a row and then both sets.

Happy Feet

One of the things that excess tension can do to you is to undermine your footwork. Feeling tense can make your feet feel like they are sticking to the court—like you have Velcro on the bottom of your shoes. In essence, your normally quick, light steps become lunging, slow, big steps. This leads to bad footwork (flatfooted), which can hurt your timing, balance, power, and consistency. To help improve footwork negatively affected by anxiety, you should think *"toes."* By staying up on your toes, you maximize the probability of taking quick, light steps, which should start to help you out of feeling tense. You want happy feet, not heavy feet.

Focus on Performance, Not Outcome

One of the real sources of anxiety is the focus on winning and losing by players. Although you hopefully always try your best to win, that does not mean you have to focus on winning. Focusing on performance (hitting your shots and doing things within your control and ability) will actually make it more likely that you will be victorious. But worrying about whether you will win or might lose, takes your focus away from what you need to do on the court, and usually produces excess anxiety and muscle tension.

Have Fun-Enjoy the Situation

When asked about retirement most tennis players cite continuing to play because they enjoy the game so much. Along these lines, when Pete Sampras was asked about retiring, since he was around 30 years old (on the old side for most professional tennis players) and his results were mediocre by the standard Sampras has set (i.e., being ranked number 1 in the world for 6 consecutive years) he simply replied, *I think I have several good years left in me. As long as I still enjoy the game and like playing, I'll continue to play.* Research has clearly revealed that enjoyment of an activity is critical for the continued long-term participation in that activity. Especially with juniors, keeping winning and losing in perspective, focusing on continually improving your game, and enjoying the competition, friendships, and other benefits of playing tennis will usually result in long-term participation.

Practice Under Stressful Circumstances

One of the best ways to prepare yourself for pressure situations is to practice under stress from time to time. It would be similar to practicing the 2-minute drill in football where coaches simulate certain circumstances (e.g., time left, score, field position etc.) and then the team needs to perform under these situations. In tennis, as you become more accustomed to playing under these conditions, you will not be as negatively affected by pressure, during actual competitions. There are all sorts of drills you can create to simulate pressure. Many coaches set up specific game situations and have players perform under these situations. For example, it might be playing a tiebreaker, serving at 5-5 in the 3rd set, trying to serve out a match 5-4 in the third, being behind 4-2 in a set, or hitting a second serve at set point. This allows you to start to develop strategies to cope with these pressure situations.

Release, Review and Reset

As noted at the outset of the book, it is what you do between points that really sets the stage for what you do during the points (since so much time- about 3/4 of the time- in a tennis match is spent between points). Karl Slaikeu and Robert Trogolo (1998) have devised a system to help players cope with anxiety and tension and quickly get them refocused between points. This basic system involves the following after every point and before the next point is played (about 25 seconds): (a) Release (followed by a STOP); (b) Review (followed by another STOP); and (c) Reset.

The Release is a letting go of the point that has just been completed. In essence, Releases are expressions of feelings and energy after a point is over and can be positive or negative. If you are feeling good then the Release will be positive such as a fist pump or some other affirmation like "way to go." If you are upset, anxious and playing poorly, the Release might take the form of yelling at yourself and telling yourself "you stink." This will typically undermine your performance and result in poor future performance. In Chapters 8 and 9 (Concentration and Self-Talk) I will discuss ways to release tension in a positive manner. But basically, positive releases are aimed at letting go of negative energy by channeling it into positive energy (see Table 6.4).

The next phase is Review, in which you think about what just happened and make plans for how to play the next point. One of the best ways to start your Review is to turn away from the net and your opponent, switch your racquet to your non-playing hand, and walk toward the back court, perhaps looking at your strings as you go. Once you have started reviewing, there are two good options: (a) what can you learn from what just happened? and (b) what can you do next? For example, say that you stayed back at the baseline and lost a long rally, yet your game plan was to come to net and force the action. This could serve as part of your review and then you could give yourself some instructions such as "get in," or "be more aggressive." This simple but quick review helps you analyze what just happened and gets you quickly refocused on what you have to do on the next point.

The last part of this between point sequence is termed *Reset* and usually refers to a pre-planned series of steps, customized to your own style of play, that will relax you (or if needed, rev you up) before the next point. This will often take the form of some sort of routine that you feel comfortable with and in which you have confidence. The key point is to make sure that you go through your routine regardless of the situation since excess stress has a way of quickening up your routine or having you forget it altogether. This issue will be discussed in more depth in the next chapter on Concentration.

Table 6.4	A Suggested Review Sequence

(1) Use specific behavior such as switching racquet to non-playing hand to start the Review

(2) Relax with a deep breath in and out (diaphragmatic breathing) as you begin the Review

(3) Walk confidently (shoulders back, head up)

(4) Look at strings, ground, or some other focal point to think

(5) Ask questions of yourself such as
• Why did I win the point?
• Why did I lose the point?
• Am I executing my game plan?
• Am I playing my opponent's weakness?
• What do I need to do next?

(6) Check your game plan to be sure you are executing it—Is it working?

(7) Consider cue words to bring focus to the Review (e.g., "be aggressive," "keep the ball deep," "hang tough," or "more topspin")

Enhancing Intensity

For most tennis players, excess anxiety and coping with this anxiety are the more typical anxiety-related problems to deal with regarding anxiety levels. But you also know that, at times, you need to pump yourself up because you might be feeling lethargic or not energized enough for match conditions. However, you don't just want to increase your activation level as this could be a different problem in and of itself. Too much arousal can be just as bad as too little as you can start to spray balls all over the place. The key is to be able to play with intensity but control. Lleyton Hewitt has this trait, as he has the ability to pump himself up (many times by pumping his fists) but stay cool, calm and focused in executing his shots. But before you can pump up and regain your intensity, you have to understand and realize the signs of being under-activated. Here are some signs of being under-activated:

• Mind constantly wandering—easily distracted.
• Feeling bored and/or uninterested.
• Heavy feeling in the legs—no bounce.
• Lack of concern for how well you are playing.
• Moving slowly—poor preparation.
• Difficulty narrowing attentional focus.
• Low energy—lack of adrenaline.

You certainly do not need to feel all of these things to be under-activated. More likely, you will probably feel a couple of these signs and symptoms when you're not really into playing. In any case, they can really undermine your game because without sufficient motivation and focus on what you are doing, it is difficult to maintain the energy level and commitment needed in a tough tennis match. These feelings can be caused by a variety of factors such as feelings of overconfidence (you're sure it's going to be an easy match and you'll win no matter what effort you put forth), feeling physically tired, not really being motivated to play since you've been playing a lot, or lack of interest (maybe it's a nice day and you are looking forward to being outside). In any case, the critical point is that the quicker you can detect and attend to these feelings, the quicker you can get yourself back on track. So here are a few suggestions for getting energized and activating your system when you are feeling slow and lethargic.

Increase Breathing Rate

We discussed slow, diaphragmatic breathing in relation to coping with excess anxiety. However, in trying to become more activated, taking short, quick breaths tends to activate or speed up the nervous system.

Physical Activity

You see lots of players jumping up and down when they are getting ready to serve or return serve. As noted earlier, other players slap their thighs or pump their fists as another physical expression of movement to become more activated. This serves to stimulate blood flow and increase heart rate which are related to higher levels of activation.

Mood Words

Many tennis players will use various "mood words" or positive statements to get themselves or keep themselves pumped up. You should choose the words that are best for you but some examples and suggestions include *hustle, tough, move, quick, fast, charge, attack, and strong.*

Act Energized

Sometimes you might not feel energetic and motivated but if you act pumped-up, you often can recapture that high energy level. We take cues from our bodies regarding how we feel, so if you keep your head up and shoulders back and walk quickly on your toes, you can often fool yourself to start feeling this way.

Upbeat Music

Something that you can do before a match to get yourself energized is to play upbeat music. Some players even do this during changeovers to enhance their mood if necessary. So take a walkman or other portable device with you and listen to your favorite upbeat music if you are feeling a little lethargic and unmotivated for an upcoming match.

CHAPTER 7

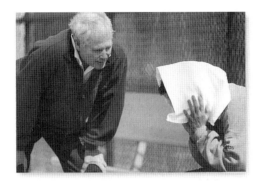

IMAGERY

Before I play a match I try to carefully rehearse in my mind what is likely to happen and how I will react in certain situations. I visualize myself playing typical points based on my opponent's style of play. I see myself hitting crisp deep shots from the baseline and coming to net if I get a weak return. This helps me prepare mentally for a match and I feel like I've already played the match before I even walk out on the court.

Chris Evert

The above quote from all-time great Chris Evert underscores the important role that imagery can play in enhancing tennis performance. This is not a technique, however, that is only used by a select few players. Research has clearly indicated that virtually all our Olympic athletes use imagery as part of their daily training regimen and approximately 90% of sport psychologists used imagery as part of their mental training programs with athletes. In fact, research has also revealed that most learners prefer input that is primarily visual, and secondarily auditory, kinesthetic and tactile. This underscores both the importance of imagery in the learning process, as well as the notion that imagery is more than just a visual activity (which will be discussed in more detail later in the chapter).

Many tennis players (myself included) have had the experience of playing at a new level after watching some great tennis players play the game. I remember going to Forest Hills (where they used to play the US Open) when I was just learning the game of tennis and watching players such as Bjorn Borg, Jimmy Connors, John Newcombe, Stan Smith, and Arthur Ashe. I used to try and visualize hitting shots like they did (of course I never did as well as them on the court), and that always seemed to help me perfect new shots and improve on shots I already had in my small repertoire. The success of Jimmy Connors and Chris Evert was directly responsible for the acceptance and eventual dominance of the two-handed backhand as many tennis pros and teachers tried to have their students copy this relatively new stroke.

Along these lines, many great players recall that they learned how to play simply by watching others. John McEnroe has said, *When I was learning to play, I just watched Rod Laver and tried to do what he did.* Ivan Lendl said he played much better after serving as a ball boy. *Being on the court so close to the players I saw things, and then I would start to do them myself.* Furthermore, when Pete Sampras switched to a one-handed backhand he watched films of Rod Laver hitting a backhand. His coach, Pete Fischer has said, *I always had an image in my mind of what a tennis player should look like. When I took Pete Sampras on as a student, I just felt I had an unlimited amount of time to make Pete into that image.* Finally, Tommy Haas' coach (who happens to be his father) instilled in him strong images of top players. So over the years, he could activate hundreds of mental images he had collected in watching the best aspects of these different players. It's obvious that players learn by watching others play and forming images in their mind about certain shots or styles of play. But what is this thing we are calling imagery from a definitional point of view?

Defining Imagery

Many terms have been used interchangeably with imagery such as visualization, mental rehearsal, and mental practice. But the key issue is that imagery refers to either creating or recreating situations in your mind. In essence, whenever you imagine yourself performing an action in the absence of physical practice, you are using imagery. So when you imagine playing your best match, really following through on all your ground strokes, or when you mentally prepare a strategy against an upcoming opponent, playing typical points in your mind, you are using imagery.

Although the term imagery implies vision or mental pictures, this is really only part of the picture. The real goal of imagery is to make the experience seem as real as possible. Therefore, for imagery to be most effective, you should include as many senses as possible. In essence, you want to really feel like you are on the tennis court. As one imagery researcher has noted, if the imagery is really powerful "the mind often does not know the difference between real and imagined stimuli." So your job is to try to include all your senses when performing imagery. An example of using all your senses in tennis is provided below.

First of all, you would use your *visual* sense to get a clear picture of your opponent hitting the ball and watching the flight of the ball as it heads toward you. Next would be your *kinesthetic* awareness (awareness of one's body movements in space) as you feel where your racquet head is on the backswing along with your transfer of weight as you move forward into the ball, Your *auditory* sense is brought into play as you hear the strings hitting the ball (there is a distinctive sound, especially with varying string tension). You can also use your auditory sense in hearing what the ball sounds like coming off your opponent's strings. You might also use your *tactile* sense, providing you feedback with how the racquet feels in your hands. Besides using all your senses, imagery can also help you create certain feelings and emotions such as confidence, anxiety, anger, or joy.

So make imagery as real as you possibly can—it will have its most potent effects if you can do this.

How Imagery Works

So how does simply visualizing a movement actually help you perform better on the tennis court? If you understand why imagery works, it should help you translate your imagery to the court more effectively. A number of different explanations for how imagery works have been developed and put forth over the years. All of these have some support although there is not one predominant approach. So these will be mentioned briefly with specific examples provided.

- *Physiological Approach.* This explanation revolves around the fact that vivid imagined events produce an innervation in your muscles that is similar to that produced by physically performing the movement. The idea is that when you vividly imagine yourself performing a movement (e.g., hitting a serve), you use similar neural pathways to those used in actually performing a serve (although not nearly to the same extent). When you physically practice serving, all you are really doing is strengthening the neural pathways that control the muscles needed to serve. One way to strengthen these neural pathways is through imagery, which really helps program your muscles to hit a perfect serve.

- *Mental Approach.* A second explanation focuses on the fact that imagery can help you understand the movement patterns necessary to perform skills, as well as execute strategies. In essence, imagery helps you form a mental blueprint of the action or strategy you have to perform. For example, your imagery would help you organize a mental plan for an upcoming opponent, familiarizing yourself with what is likely to occur, and your shot selection and execution in response to these potential situations.

- *Psychological Skills.* A third way that imagery has been hypothesized to work is through the development of psychological skills. Recent research has shown that imagery can have an effect on such psychological states as confidence, anxiety, concentration, anger, and motivation. So, even though you might have lost several times in a row to a particular opponent and might lack confidence, through imagery you can increase your confidence, because you can see yourself playing well and beating this opponent.

Types of Imagery

When tennis players image, they usually do it from either an internal or external perspective. The differences in these two types of imagery will be discussed below, regarding the form that they take and their effectiveness on enhancing performance.

Internal Imagery

Internal imagery refers to imagining performing a skill from your own eyes. In essence, you could only see what you normally would see, as it's like having a camera on your head which took pictures of all the things you could see while executing the skill. For example, when imaging hitting a tennis serve from an internal perspective, you would see the racquet and ball in your hand during the ready position, your opponent, where in the service box you want to hit the ball, the ball toss and contact point. However, you would not be able to see your backswing or anything else outside of your normal vision.

External Imagery

External imagery involves visualizing a movement as if you were watching yourself on a VCR. Since you are watching yourself, as opposed to actually doing the movement (as in internal imagery), you could see not only the things you would normally see, but you could see your backswing, weight transfer and the arch in your back, since you are taking the perspective of a spectator.

Internal or External: That is the Question

The question then becomes, which of these two perspectives results in better performance or other outcomes (e.g., staying more relaxed on the court, enhancing confidence, staying focused). At first, researchers felt that internal imagery would be superior, since it was thought that players could get more of a feeling for the movement when they were actually doing it in their mind. But research has revealed that both perspectives can be effective. What appears to be more important is getting a vivid, controllable image (we'll discuss this a little later in the chapter). So don't be overly concerned with imagery perspective as either one will work. Some situations might be better served using an external perspective, especially if you are trying to change a stroke and need to see clearly what you are doing correctly or incorrectly. Therefore, external imagery might be particularly effective to drill specific shots or techniques such as your service, and this visual perspective corresponds well with video-taped pictures. Other situations might just require strengthening the neural patterns of the skill or setting up a game plan for a specific opponent and an internal perspective may be more beneficial. In addition, also use internal imagery especially when you have to make adjustments in response to changes from your opponent.

Imagery Evaluation

Research has clearly indicated that one of the most important factors affecting the success of imagery (if not the most important) is how skillful an individual is at imaging. In essence, as has been emphasized throughout this book, imagery is a skill (like other psychological skills) and needs to be practiced and learned like physical skills. Therefore, some of you might be pretty good at it (or at least several aspects of imaging) or have practiced a great deal while others may never have done it before or have trouble even getting an image. But before you start practicing, you need to know what your strengths and weaknesses are regarding your imagery ability. In addition, you should know what kinds of imagery you use as well as how frequently you use them and how effective they are for you. To assess how well you use your senses while imaging, please complete the inventory in Table 7.1. For those areas in which you scored lower, you might be particularly sensitive and pay close attention to what's happening on the court. So if you scored low, for example, on auditory imagery, you might pay particular attention to the sounds you hear on court, so that you might incorporate them into your next imagery training session.

Table 7.1	Vividness of Imagery Questionnaire

As you complete this questionnaire (adapted from Martens (1982) remember that imagery involves more than just seeing something in your mind. Vivid images include not only visualizing, but also experiencing different senses–seeing, hearing, feeling, and smelling. In addition, you may also experience moods, affect or states of mind.

 Below you will read descriptions of four different situations in tennis. You will be asked to imagine each situation as vividly as possible trying to make the image as real as you can. Then you will be asked to rate your imagery on the following dimensions.

A. Visual (sight) 1 = No image present to 5 = Extremely clear and vivid image
B. Auditory (sounds) 1= No sounds heard to 5 = Extremely clear sounds
C. Kinesthetic (feelings) 1 = No feelings associated with the movement to 5 = Extremely clear sensations of making the movement
D. Mood (Emotions) 1 = No feelings present to 5 = Extremely clear feelings

After you read each general description, think of a specific example of it (e.g., the skill, people involved, the place, the time). Next, close your eyes and take a few deep breaths to become as relaxed as you can. Keep your eyes closed for about one minute as you try to imagine the situation as vividly as possible.

Practicing Alone
Select one specific skill such as hitting a forehand, backhand, or serve. Now imagine yourself performing this shot at a place where you normally practice without anyone else present. Close your eyes for a minute and try to see yourself at this place performing the skill. See yourself, hear the sounds, feel your body performing the movements and be aware of your state of mind or mood.

Table 7.1	Vividness of Imagery Questionnaire cont.

How vivid was your image? (use the 1-5 scale provided on previous page)

A. Visual _____   C. Kinesthetic _____

B. Auditory _____   D. Mood _____

Practicing With Others

You are doing the same activity but now you are practicing the skill with your coach and your teammates present. See yourself making a mistake as well as a great shot that everyone notices. For about a minute, imagine the situation as vividly as possible along the four dimensions discussed previously.

How vivid was your image? (use the 1-5 scale on previous page)

A. Visual _____   C. Kinesthetic _____

B. Auditory _____   D. Mood _____

Watching a Teammate or Competitor

Think of a teammate or competitor performing a specific shot unsuccessfully and then successfully in a match. For example, imagine a double fault followed by an ace or your teammate netting an easy volley and then putting a volley away for a winner. Take about a minute and imagine the situation as vividly as possible using the four dimensions

How vivid was your image? (use the 1-5 scale provided on previous page)

A. Visual _____   C. Kinesthetic _____

B. Auditory _____   D. Mood _____

Competitive Performance

Imagine yourself performing in a match. You are playing extremely well and the spectators and your teammates are showing their appreciation. Take about a minute and imagine the situation as vividly as possible using the four dimensions provided on previous page

How vivid was your image? (use the 1-5 scale provided on previous page).

A. Visual _____   C. Kinesthetic _____

B. Auditory _____   D. Mood _____

Scoring

Now let's determine your imagery scores and see what they mean. First, add the ratings for your answers to part A for each of the four scenarios. Then add the scores for each of your four answers for Parts B, C, and D. Record them below and then add the total.

Table 7.1	Vividness of Imagery Questionnaire cont.

A. Visual _____ + _____ + _____ + _____ = _____
B. Auditory _____ + _____ + _____ + _____ = _____
C. Kinesthetic _____ + _____ + _____ + _____ = _____
D. Mood _____ + _____ + _____ + _____ = _____

Each of the three dimensions could have totaled a maximum score of 20 and a minimum score of 4. The closer you came to 20 on each dimension, the more skill you are currently demonstrating in that dimension of imagery. Lower scores suggest that you should work on those aspects of your imagery.

Basic Imagery Training

Regardless of how well you did on the imagery questionnaire, imagery is a skill and should be practiced. Great tennis players continue to practice their best shots so that they can get even better or at least maintain their level of proficiency. The same can be said for the skill of imagery. You can take the information from the test you just took, to provide feedback regarding specific areas on which to concentrate. But the basic imagery training provided here will focus on vividness and controllability.

Vividness

As discussed earlier, your imagery should be as vivid as possible and employ as many senses as possible. This will maximize the transfer to actual performance. Your evaluation from Table 7.1, basically focused on the vividness of your images. Remember, the body can't tell the difference between real and vividly imagined experiences. Here are a few sample exercises to help build the vividness of your imagery.

Your Living Room

Imagine that you are at home in your living room. Place yourself somewhere in the living room that allows you to see the rest of the room. Look around and take in all the details. What do you see? Notice the shape and texture of the furniture. What is the temperature like? What sounds do you hear? Is there any movement in the air? What odors do you smell? Use all of your senses to take it all in.

Positive Performance of a Tennis Skill

Select a particular shot and visualize yourself performing it perfectly. I will use the serve as an example but you can use whatever shot you'd like (or try imagery with a variety of shots). Start by seeing yourself in the ready position, looking at your opponent in the service court, and then pick the spot where you want the serve to go. See and feel how you start the service motion and release the ball at the perfect height, the toss going just where you want. Feel your back arch and your shoulders stretch, as you take the racquet back behind your head. Feel your weight start to transfer forward and your arm and racquet reach high to contact the ball at just the right height and angle. Feel your wrist snap as you explode into the ball. Hear the racquet contact the ball noticing different sounds for different types of shots (e.g., slice, topspin, flat). Now see and feel the follow-through with your weight coming completely forward. The ball goes exactly where you wanted it to, forcing a high floating return from your opponent. You close into the net and put the ball away with a firm cross-court volley.

Recall a Positive Performance

Recall a time when you performed extremely well. Your visualization should cover sight, sound, feelings and mood (affect). In visual recall, imagine how you look when you're playing well as opposed to playing poorly. These typically differ substantially from the way you walk, carry your shoulders to how you swing the racquet. A confident tennis player often looks different on the outside, just as he or she feels different on the inside. View videotapes of successful performances to help create vivid images.

Next, focus on the sounds you hear when you are playing well. Especially important is the internal dialogue you have with yourself (this self-talk will be discussed in more detail in Chapter 9). There is often an internal silence that accompanies your best performances. Listen to it. What is your internal dialogue like? What are you saying to yourself and how are you saying it? What about other sounds like the strings hitting the ball, spectators, and airplanes overhead. Recreate all these sounds as vividly as possible.

For kinesthetic recall, recreate clearly in your mind all the bodily sensations you have when playing well. How do your hands and feet feel? Do you have a feeling of quickness, looseness, speed or intensity in your body? How does the racquet feel in your hand? How do the different strokes feel? Focus on the bodily sensations that are associated with playing well.

For recalling mood, think about what you were thinking and feeling when you were playing well. When we play well, we usually feel confident, have low levels of anxiety, are focused, are not angry, and are motivated. Try to incorporate your feelings into imagery when playing well.

Controllability

Another aspect to successful imagery is making sure that you control your images so that they do what you want them to do. Some players I have worked with have had difficulty controlling their image. For example, players may visualize their serve going into the net or their angled volleys just drifting wide. You want to see your body hit great shots, not make unforced errors and double faults. The following exercises are designed to help control your images.

Controlling Performance

Imagine hitting a stroke that has given you trouble in the past (maybe it's an overhead, a second serve, return of serve or reflex volley). Notice what you are doing wrong. Now, make some correction to improve the performance of that skill. See and feel your movements and watch the ball go exactly where you want it to go. For example, see and feel yourself hitting a backhand passing shot cross court, just out of the reach of your opponent or hitting a return of serve at your opponent's feet, causing an error.

Controlling Performance in a Difficult Match

Picture yourself in a difficult match, one in which you have had trouble in the past. It might be serving for the match, hitting a second serve under pressure, getting behind early, or missing a critical shot at break point. Put yourself in these situations and then see yourself staying focused and calm and hitting great shots. For example, you might picture yourself serving for the match and continuing to do the things that got you there—good first serves, deep, consistent ground strokes, and being aggressive on short balls.

Recovering from a Mistake in a Critical Situation

Imagine yourself in a situation in which you have just made a mistake (e.g., missed an easy volley, doubled faulted, missed a routine ground stroke). This is a critical situation such as break point or game point. Try to recreate the situation, especially the emotions and feelings that flooded you after making the mistake. You might feel angry, frustrated, tense, or lacking in confidence after making this error. For example, if you felt tense, you could use one of the anxiety management strategies discussed in Chapter 5 and feel the tension drain out of your body. Again, the focus is on controlling what you see, hear, and feel in your imagery.

Imagery Training

Thus far, you have been exposed to the basic tenets of imagery, as well as some imagery evaluation and basic imagery training in vividness and controllability. Now, I will provide you with some guidelines for setting up an individualized imagery training program for yourself or your team. It is important to remember that imagery programs need to be tailored for the individual based on their needs, interests and abilities as a tennis player. The program need not be complex or cumbersome, but should fit nicely into your daily routine. Pick out the things that make the most sense to you and start with these as a basis for your program. Other things can be added as you go along.

Start in a Relaxed State

Research has revealed that imagery preceded by relaxation is more effective than imagery alone. So make sure that prior to every imagery session you try to relax by using one of the techniques discussed in Chapter 5 such as deep breathing, progressive relaxation or any technique that works for you. This is only to be done for a short period (a couple of minutes) before getting started with your imagery session. Relaxing helps imaging because it helps you forget your daily worries and hassles and focuses your concentration on the task at hand. In addition, a relaxed state will result in more powerful imagery, because it won't have to compete with other events.

Have Realistic Expectations and Motivation

In working with many tennis players over the years, I have run across a couple of problems relating to expectations and motivation. On the one hand, there are some players who believe that imagery will make them better players overnight and will magically transform them into the player of their dreams. Certainly imagery can help improve your performance and attitude on the court. But it won't make you a Serena Williams or Lleyton Hewitt if you only have average skill.

The other problem I often face is that some players simply don't believe in imagery, as they feel only physical practice can help their games. Such negative thinking often undermines the potential effectiveness of imagery and imagery is practiced in a haphazard fashion. Remember that imagery requires the same type of motivation and commitment as working on physically changing your service motion or backhand. So expect that imagery will help and if you stay dedicated and motivated to your imagery training program, your efforts will be rewarded in the future.

Image as Realistically as Possible

I can't emphasize enough the idea that your images should be as real life as possible. Thus the use of as many senses as appropriate, is essential as is the ability to control your images. The old computer saying, "garbage in, garbage out" certainly applies here. If your mind-body software is producing flawed images of technique or negative emotional states, it's unlikely that your game will improve (this is where your imagery evaluation and training should be helpful). It might be a good idea to schedule a lesson or two with your tennis coach or teaching professional for a technical check-up before you embark on your imagery program. Also, remember that in addition to creating vivid and controllable images (exercises were provided previously), make sure to include the psychological states that you would like to experience on the court. Thus your imagery should include feelings of confidence, attentional control, feelings of optimal arousal and any other psychological states that enhance your performance.

Positive/Coping Focus

Research has indicated that focusing your imagery on the positive, will be most helpful to your game. Generally speaking, most of the time you should see yourself playing flawless but realistic tennis. Create scenarios in which you remain ideally balanced, focused, hit the ball in front of you, and are winning challenging points. If you want to improve your serve and volley game, you might visualize yourself hitting strong, deep, and accurate serves, following it up with a split step inside the baseline, a crisp deep volley, and then closing down on the net for a put-away volley.

However, no player is perfect, and we all make mistakes. In fact, the player with the least unforced errors, will usually win the match. So in your imagery, you want to see yourself occasionally making an error or experiencing a negative emotion. In essence, in the spirit of making imagery realistic, you'll want to see yourself overcome poor execution of a shot or poor shot selection. This type of imagery is known as coping imagery, since you try to see yourself effectively coping with a negative event.

It is especially important in tennis to be able to leave a missed shot behind you and go on to the next point with a clear mind (this is difficult in part due to the 25-30 seconds between every point in tennis). There are different ways to accomplish this, but imagery is certainly one effective way of coping with mistakes. For example, imagine serving at 5-4, 40-30 in the first set (you have a set point) and you miss your first serve. But now you use your imagery to visualize your pre-serve routine, taking a deep breath before serving, and then serving a strong second serve with lots of topspin, which gives you a large margin for error. You go on to win the point and with it the set. Or maybe you missed an easy volley, passing shot, or return of serve at an important point in the match. This might normally be accompanied by getting mad and frustrated on the next point(s). In your imagery, you can see yourself recovering from this mistake, staying calm and focused, and then executing the shots in your next point to perfection. In fact, research with Olympic athletes (Greenleaf, Gould, & Dieffenbach, 2001) has found that preparing for and coping with mistakes and unusual events was the most important discriminator between athletes' performing over their potential (won a medal but not expected to win) and those performing under their potential (expected to win a medal but did not). There may be one or two situations or errors from which you have trouble recovering; imagery is a perfect tool to practice coping effectively with these problem areas.

Image in Real Time

Your imagery will be most helpful if you image in real time rather than in slow or fast motion. Players have a tendency to image too fast (faster than the actual time it takes to perform the movement), so it's important to slow down and image in real time. This is an outgrowth of keeping your images as real life as possible. It also helps the muscle memory to remember, since you are imprinting the neurological system in the way and timing it is typically done. For example, let's say that you have a pre-serve routine that takes 15 seconds (we'll discuss routines in Chapter 8). If you want to image this routine, then it should take 15 seconds in your imagery, not 10 or 20 seconds. You might have someone actually time how long it takes to play out different points or how long you usually take between points, as this will also help you get a sense of real time.

Image Execution and Outcome

In working with tennis players over the years, I have found that they often tend to imagine the outcome of a shot but not the execution or vice versa. It is important to visualize both how you want to perform the skill as well as the outcome of it. So, in hitting a deep crisp volley, you might want to imagine your body position, court position, positioning of your racquet, footwork, and any other relevant cues, but also image exactly where you want the ball to go in the court.

Videotapes/Audiotapes

In consulting with tennis players, I have found that they often can get a clear, vivid image of their teammates or frequent opponents, but have trouble imagining themselves. This is because it is difficult to visualize something you have never seen before. To overcome this obstacle, simply have someone make a video of you, including all your strokes and movements from side to side as well as up and back. If you are more of a beginner, you might want to model some of the strokes of the great champions (you might want to do this even if you are not a beginner). Oftentimes, seeing themselves on video for the first time is quite eye-opening for tennis players. For example, I remember when I first saw a video of my service motion and my first comment was, "is that me?" But it really helped me understand and visualize what I was doing (or not doing) and allowed me to get a much clearer picture of myself and improve my serve.

If you can, splice the film and pick out only your best shots and then duplicate them repeatedly on the tape. This will give you a better picture of how you look when you are hitting the ball well and is a great way to initiate imagery prior to playing a match. Some top tennis players like Andre Agassi have made up a "highlight video" of themselves playing well in particular situations during competitions, as well as getting the feeling of winning these matches and events. The edited highlights of these best ever moments are then set to the player's favorite motivational music. This type of video could be used with your own imagery to boost confidence and motivation, or it may simply enhance the clarity and vividness of your images. In addition, looking at a video may help locate a particular problem in stroke production. Then in your imagery (as well as on the court), you can correct this technical problem and image the correct stroke technique.

Besides using video tapes to help your imagery, you could also use audio tapes. Although there are many commercial audio tapes available, these tapes are usually not specific enough for each tennis player. In essence, audio tapes need to be individualized to fit the needs of each and every player. You could make a tape up for yourself or have a coach make it up for you. In either case, make sure that the tape includes specific verbal cues that are familiar and meaningful to you, including specific responses to various match situations that may arise during a match. I will supply you with a sample, guided imagery scenario (mentally preparing for a match) in Table 7.2, but you would likely modify it somewhat to fit your own particular needs (see Table 7.3 for guidelines for developing your personal imagery tape). Optimally, you would watch this at home right before leaving for a match or maybe on site in a locker room or other quiet place.

Table 7.2	Imagery Script (Preparing for a Match)

You step out on the court to warm up and your feet feel light and bouncy. Your ground strokes are fluid and easy, yet powerful. You feel the short back swing and nice follow-through on your shots. You are moving around the court freely and effortlessly, getting to all of your opponent's shots. You warm up your volley and overhead and everything feels good. Your contact point on your volleys is out in front of you and you are anticipating well. You feel a nice stretch on the back of your arm and in your lower back as you go back to hit some overheads. They are clean and right in the center of the racquet. As you warm up your serve you feel that your motion is fluid, your ball toss is consistent and you're really reaching out and transferring your weight into the ball. The ball is hitting the spots in the service box that you are aiming for, using a variety of serves, spins and speeds.

You now see yourself starting the match serving and getting right into the flow of the match. You visualize some strong serves where your opponent can only just get the ball back to the mid court and you decisively put the ball away with short, topspin, angled strokes. Your next point is a long rally from baseline to baseline. You see yourself keeping the ball deep and hitting it firmly but yet with a good margin for error. Finally, your opponent hits a short ball and you come in and slice it deep to the backhand corner. Your opponent tries a down the line passing shot but you guess right and are right there to hit a short cross court volley winner. You finish the game with a big serve down the middle of the "t" for an ace. This game gets you off to a fast start and gets your adrenaline flowing and concentration focused on the match. As you get ready to walk out onto the court, you are feeling relaxed and confident. You can't wait to start hitting the ball.

Practice Strategies as Well as Strokes

Although most players tend to focus on hitting certain shots in their imagery, it is equally as effective to imagine the execution of different strategies against different opponents. Brad Gilbert in his book *Winning Ugly*, talks a lot about knowing the tendencies of your opponents by scouting them and noting what they like or don't like to do in different situations (especially

Table 7.3   Guidelines for Developing Your Personal Imagery Tape

Format of Your Tape

- *Music or not*—If you use music, make sure it puts you into a confident state, not too pumped up (hard driving music) or too relaxed (soft music).
- *Whose voice*—Use your own voice if possible and speak slowly and clearly. Use someone else's voice if your voice makes you nervous.

Include All Senses

- *Vision*—What does the court look like? What does the scene around the court look like? Do you see colors? Do you see your opponent or the audience?
- *Hearing*—What sounds do you hear throughout the match?
- *Touch*—How does the racquet feel in your hand?
- *Kinesthetic*—How do your arm and back feel during the serve?
- *Smell*—Are there any food smells or other smells around the courts?

Four Phases of Your Tape

- *Relaxation*—Include a relaxation phase of deep breathing, counting the breaths in and out. Do this for a minute or two.
- *Before Your Match*—Go through your pre-match routine (especially as you arrive at the court). Make sure you are feeling relaxed, confident, and focused. Go over your game plan.
- *During Your Match*—Imagine points being played out and see yourself playing great tennis. You are feeling strong and focused and use all your senses to get the feel of the match. See yourself playing the kind of points that you would like to play. You are carrying out your game plan to perfection.
- *After the Match*—After seeing yourself play great tennis, take a moment to feel the success. Get a vivid image of what it feels like to play at the top of your game. Slowly take some deep breaths and become more alert as you conclude your imagery.

when the pressure is on). Imagery is a good way to prepare for players once you know some of their strengths, weaknesses, and tendencies. With this information, you could play out different points in your mind, mentally trying to hit different shots from different positions on the court. For example, if your opponent is a net rusher, you might see yourself making a good low return so that your opponent needs to volley up, giving you a chance for a passing shot. But you also know that your opponent likes to close down on the net. So in your imagery, you visualize a perfect offensive lob over his backhand side that is just out of his reach. You can play out in your mind different types of points and shots that you expect to see in the actual match. In this way, you are ready for these situations and have started to program your body to react in certain ways.

When to Use Imagery

Recent research has found that imagery is used in a variety of situations although players tend to use it before competition in preparing for a match. But I would encourage that imagery be practiced in a variety of settings and used in different circumstances to enhance its positive effects on performance, affect, and thinking. I would also suggest that you use imagery during practice for about 10-15 minutes on a consistent basis, so that you can better learn the skill of imagery and apply it to match situations. Tennis players have confirmed that using imagery consistently helps them form more vivid and controllable images as they learn the best way to use imagery to help their particular situation.

Before and After Practices

As noted on several occasions, imagery is a mental skill and thus needs to be practiced on a regular basis to gain maximum benefits. One way to learn and improve upon your imagery skills is to consistently practice both before and after practice. This could be done with a coach taking you through some imagery before practice, or you could use the imagery script provided in this chapter (or you can modify the script to fit your needs). This will help warm up the nervous system to play tennis at top efficiency level. It's important that imagery be seen as part of regular practice and not as an "add on." In this way tennis players will see it as just another part of their training regimen.

It is also appropriate to use imagery after physical practice, because after working out, you should have the feel of your strokes and movement fresh in your mind. This will help you create imagery that is very detailed and clear and uses all senses, like we had discussed earlier. You should also be able to "feel" the movement even better since this feeling should be etched in your muscles from the physical workout. The key is to do this for 10 minutes or so a regular basis so that you will maximize the positive effects of imagery and improve your skill of imagery at the same time.

Before and After Competition

Our research (Weinberg, Butt, Knight, & Burke, 2003) has clearly shown that the most popular time for using imagery is before competition (especially a big competition which is seen as important). There is nothing wrong with this (in fact, I would encourage it) as long as you have worked on developing your imagery skills during practice or at other times. Before competition, imagery can help you focus if you review in your mind exactly what you want to do, including your game plan for the upcoming match. Our research has also shown that players particularly image difficult, pressure-filled situations so that they are ready for them when they occur. In addition, you can go over your strokes and start to get the feeling of hitting different shots before going out and warming-up. As noted earlier, several professional tennis players consistently prepare for competition using imagery, although the timing tends to be individualized, with some preferring to do it right before coming out on the court, while others image an hour or two before competition. What's probably most important is that imagery fit comfortably into your pre-match routine (we'll discuss this in Chapter 8) and it should not be forced or rushed. Furthermore, you might choose to use imagery at two or three different times prior to a match. If this is the case, then one session (lasting about 10 minutes) could focus on your strategy and the other on stroke production, getting a feel for your strokes. The pre-match possibilities for imagery are endless and ultimately, depend on personal preference.

An often overlooked time to use imagery is right after competition. At this time, most players tend to be focused on match outcome, and forget to realize that this is a great time to employ imagery. Like after practice, the feeling of your shots are still with you and the strategy of the match is also fresh in your mind. So this time could be used to remember what you did well and recapture that image and feeling with your visualization. In addition, you can also replay unsuccessful shots and points, imagining yourself performing successfully or choosing different shots or strategy. For instance, I recently played a tournament match in which I lost in a closely contested 3rd set tiebreaker. On match point I missed one of my favorite shots—an inside–out forehand—and I had missed this shot several times throughout the match. So I decided to use some imagery and practice this particular shot over and over again. In my next match, a couple of days later, I hit this shot exceedingly well, including during several pressure (break) points, which helped me to win the match. I should note that I also imaged this shot prior to playing as part of my pre-match routine. But the takeaway point is to employ imagery after matches as well as before matches.

During Breaks in the Action

Due to the start and stop nature of tennis, it is possible to use imagery between points to get ready for the next point since every point begins with a serve or service return. So using imagery at these junctures can help you prepare for the next shot and point. Of course you have to practice your imagery first before you can use it as part of a service or service return routine. We will discuss service and service return imagery in the next chapter (Chapter 8).

The other time where there is a break in the action is during changeovers which can be about 60-90 seconds. This is a time when most players try to catch their breath and try to get ready for the next game(s). This is a perfect time to use imagery to get yourself ready for the next game or so. So after you have gotten a drink and caught your breath, sit down and take a few seconds to get ready for the next couple of games. If you are serving, you can visualize hitting strong and accurate serves and following them up with crisp ground strokes. If you're returning, you can picture yourself being on your toes and ready, and hitting the ball in front of you with a short backswing, keeping the ball low at the opponent's feet as that person rushes the net. Or you might visualize strategy (especially if playing on a slower surface like clay), seeing yourself hit a variety of shots as you methodically set up the point. In any case, imagery is a useful tool to use when there is a little time between points, as many players do not use this time efficiently or effectively. So practice your imagery, so you can use it during a match.

During Personal Time

The other time and place to practice your imagery would be outside of the practice or match situation, during your personal time. This might likely be at home, but could be accomplished at any appropriate quiet place. So set aside 10-15 minutes per day (it's best if you do this at a set time so you can have it as a routine) to practice various parts of your imagery whether it be vividness, controllability, particular strokes, or match strategy. Sometimes it's even best to use imagery at home before practices or matches since there is not always a good place to image right before practice or competitions. In any case, personal time is a great time to practice your imagery, as you can determine the best time and place to set up your practice.

Recovering From Injury

One of the most appropriate times to use imagery is when you are injured or somehow unable to physically practice or play. Injured tennis players have used imagery to rehearse performance as well as the emotions they anticipate experiencing upon return to competition. In one study, Ieleva and Orlick, (1991) found that positive images of healing were related to faster recovery times. There are also many anecdotal reports of athletes using imagery when injured, thus keeping the neurological connections working until their subsequent return to action. Here, use of videotapes would be particularly important as this would help keep the images very vivid and realistic.

CHAPTER 8

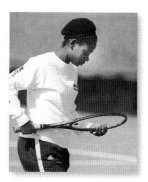

CONCENTRATION

You can hardly hear a player talk about a tennis match without mentioning "focus," whether he was really focused or whether he lost focus during the match. When player's talk about focus, they are really talking about concentration or attentional focus.

The importance of concentration is underscored by the following comment of Chris Evert:

> *Ninety percent of my game is mental. It's my concentration that got me so far in tennis I won't even call a friend the day of a match. I'm scared of disrupting my concentration. I don't allow any competition with tennis.*

Although you probably have an idea what concentration is all about, let's start out by defining it, especially in terms of tennis, so we can start with a common language.

What is Concentration?

In Chapter 2, we discussed the notion of optimal performance, and one of the critical states was that of complete concentration. Concentration boils down to how frequently you think about something and the nature of those thoughts. Michael Johnson, world record holder in the 400 meter dash and Olympic Gold Medalist, describes his single-minded focus and concentration during a race.

> *I have learned to cut all unnecessary thoughts on the track. I simply concentrate. I concentrate on the tangible—on the track, on the race, on the blocks, on the things I have to do. The crowd fades away and other athletes disappear and now it's just me and this one lane.*

Sometimes being totally focused seems to mean that you appear to have nothing going on at all in your head. In essence, your mind is clear of all distractions and is totally focused on the here and now. This is seen in Pete Sampras' comment during his 1999 Wimbledon championship run when serving at match point (where he hit a second serve ace). *There was absolutely nothing going on in my mind at that time.* This is reminiscent of the focused concentration discussed as part of peak performance states in Chapter 2. So what is this thing we call *concentration* (or at least its component parts)?

Focusing on Relevant Cues

In terms of sport psychology, concentration can be seen as consisting of two different but related aspects. First, is the ability to focus on the relevant cues in your environment. For a tennis player the most obvious (although sometimes overlooked) is watching the ball. Although this seems so basic and straightforward, it is often the undoing of many tennis players. Specifically, many players focus in the general direction of the ball but don't really focus on the ball itself. Another important cue is the opponent's racquet work, movements, and court positioning before they hit the ball, in order to help anticipate the direction, speed and placement of the shot. So if an opponent is deep in the backhand side and takes his racquet head back high and starts to turn his body early, you might anticipate a slice crosscourt return. We also cue ourselves before hitting the ball with words such as *bend, racquet back, firm wrist, follow-through,* and *forward.*

Interestingly, it is not actually playing points that create as many problems with attentional focus as between points. While we are playing points, there are relevant cues (like those discussed above) that often occupy our mind. But between points (and sometimes during points), there are a host of irrelevant cues that compete for our attention. These can range from previously missed shots, antics of our opponent, crowd noises, plans for the evening, a bad line call, what happened the day before, a business meeting, or anything else the mind can conjure up. Focusing on these between points, makes it more likely that they will take up some of our attentional focus during the points. So your job is to keep these irrelevant thoughts from entering your mind, in order to free up your focus to attend to only the relevant cues in your environment. Top players such as Patrick Rafter, Lindsay Davenport, Lleyton Hewitt, and Venus Williams (just to name a few), have the ability to stay focused on the relevant cues during a match despite what is going on around them. Martina Hingis (who generally stays focused) lost her focus completely when arguing over a line call in the French Open final against Steffi Graf. After winning the first set, Hingis became completely unraveled after this incident and went on to lose the match and Championship. The problem that often occurs when you lose your concentration and focus on irrelevant cues, is that you tend to do that for several points (or even several games) and this really can undermine your performance.

Maintaining Concentration

The other aspect to concentration has to do with the ability to maintain that focus over time. A tennis match can easily take a couple of hours (or more for five set matches in the men's Grand Slams) and one break in concentration can often mean the difference. A quote by all-time great Bjorn Borg underscores this point.

> *Very often in a tennis match, you can point to just one game where for a couple of points you lost concentration and didn't do the right thing, and the difference in the match will be right there.*
>
> *(Tarshis, 1977, p. 21)*

Let's take a practical example of a small lapse in concentration being critical in a match. You are holding serve easily, whereas your opponent is struggling but still holding on to serve. Then at 4-4, 30-30 you are serving and you have a high forehand putaway volley. But just as you are about to hit the ball you notice your opponent is moving in the direction in which you intended to hit the ball. At the last instant you change your mind and try to go behind your opponent but miss the line by a few inches. You immediately become mad at yourself for taking your eye off the ball and missing such as easy shot. You are still mad as you serve and try to hit a big serve only to hit a fault. You then go for a big second serve and miss again for a break in serve. Your opponent is more confident after this break and easily holds serve for the set. You are still thinking about the easy volley you missed throughout the game and don't really concentrate on breaking back.

Although this has been stated often, concentration is a psychological skill that needs to be practiced on a regular basis. All time great Rod Laver makes this point.

> *There's no secret to building concentration. It's something you develop the same way you develop other parts of your game. The mistake most club players make is that they don't practice concentration while they're practicing their strokes. If your mind is going to wander during practice, it's going to do the same in a match. What I used to do was to force myself to concentrate more as soon as I'd feel myself getting tired, because that's usually when your concentration starts to fall off.*
>
> *(Tarshis, 1977, p. 31)*

This quote highlights the point that concentration can be developed through deliberate practice. Rod Laver and his coaches were really aware that if you don't work on developing concentration in practice, you can't automatically turn on your concentration during a competitive match. This is particularly the case when you become fatigued as your mind is more likely to wander at this time in a match. This is a mistake that many junior and club players make, believing that it's only important to concentrate in the matches. But there are things you can do on and off the court to help build your concentration skills and these will be discussed later in the chapter. So why is it so hard to maintain concentration in a competitive match?

Difficulty in Maintaining Concentration

You wouldn't think it would be too difficult to maintain concentration throughout a competitive match, but in fact it is. The difficulty could be traced to two primary factors: (a) the nature of the mind and (b) the nature of the game of tennis.

Regarding the workings of the mind, your attentional focus is typically dependent on your motivation and intensity or importance of the specific event/stimuli in question. The principle is basically that the more intense the stimuli, the less motivation you need to maintain concentration, whereas the less intense the stimuli the more motivation you need to sustain your concentration. That is why it is typically easier to sustain motivation against a tough opponent in a close match (important situation), than against a lesser opponent whom you have beaten several times previously, and you're up 4-1 in the first set. In the latter example, you might be thinking already about your next opponent or what you were going to do that evening. So now it is 4-1 and your motivation and intensity will typically be lowered as will your concentration (unfortunately for you, the concentration of your opponent will likely be heightened if he or she is a good competitor).

In essence, you bring to the tennis court a mind that is always receptive to things other than relevant tennis cues. It is your job to keep the mind focused on your tennis game and try to disregard other competing thoughts. Remember that equal skills and challenges is one of the critical aspects of getting into a Flow state as discussed in Chapter 2. So when, for example, challenges are too easy for your skills, your mind will more likely wander and your concentration will be compromised.

The second reason that maintaining concentration is so difficult, is due to the start and stop nature of tennis (as noted at the outset of this chapter). More specifically, statistics reveal that the average point lasts 8-12 seconds, yet you have up to 30 seconds between points. In a two-hour match, then, only about 40 minutes are actually spent playing tennis. It is this "dead" time that taxes concentration because of the numerous distractions competing for our attentional focus. So what we do with all this "down" time makes it difficult to maintain concentration (a similar but even more serious problem is all the dead time in golf between shots). But attentional focus takes a variety of forms as seen below.

Types of Attentional Focus

Research has clearly found that attentional focus can vary across two dimensions: *width* and *direction*. Width of attention can vary from very broad to very narrow. For example in tennis a broad focus would be necessary in doubles to watch the movements of your partner as well as opponents. A narrow focus would be typical of tennis players who focus exclusively on the ball in preparation for their shot.

Attention can also vary in direction ranging from internal to external. External attention would be characterized by focusing outward on the external environment like the ball or movements of your opponent. An internal focus means focusing on your own thoughts and feelings such as "I need to be more aggressive and come to net when I get a short ball" or "I need to keep my service toss more out in front of me." This focus on width and direction of attention results in four different basic attentional styles displayed in Table 8.1.

Table 8.1	Direction of Attention	
Width of Attention	**External**	**Internal**
Broad	Used to rapidly assess a situation (doubles exchange at net)	Used to analyze and plan (e.g., developing a game plan against a tough opponent)
Narrow	Used to focus exclusively on one or two external cues (e.g., watching the ball)	Used to mentally rehearse an upcoming performance or control an emotional state (e.g., mentally rehearse the tennis serve or focus on taking a deep breath before serving to relax)

Changing Attentional Focus

Besides knowing the different types of attentional focus, it is important to know how quickly this attention must change in a tennis match and what type of attentional focus is appropriate for different situations on the tennis court. Let's take a situation where you are playing an opponent who beat you last time because of his aggressive play at the net. To develop a game plan requires a *broad-internal* focus as you decide that you need to be more aggressive and approach the net on short balls that are hit around the service line. As you go out on the court and warm-up, you change to a *broad-external* focus taking in important environmental information such as the wind, sun and temperature, as well as the speed of the playing surface and opponent's strokes and movement. After you have quickly assessed the situation, you start focusing on yourself which requires a *narrow-internal* focus. This might mean focusing on your strokes, feeling loose and relaxed, getting your timing down, making good solid contact with the ball, feeling light on your feet, as well as attending to other kinesthetic cues to hone your strokes. As you finish your warm-up and get ready to begin the match, you start to narrow your focus by watching the ball and getting tuned into the match, which requires a *narrow-external* focus. As you continue to play, you will probably change from being more internally-focused between points and externally-focused within points. The key is to have the ability to shift your attentional focus at appropriate times so that you have the right focus for the right situation. We'll discuss this proper focus more throughout the chapter.

Attentional Problems

Many tennis players I have worked with have had problems concentrating for the duration of a match. Usually, these concentration problems are caused by inappropriate attentional focus. As shown by the extensive research of Jackson and Csikszentmihalyi (1999) interviewing elite athletes, worries and irrelevant thoughts can cause athletes to withdraw their concentration "beam" from what they were doing to what they hope will not happen. In essence, they are not focusing on the proper cues; rather they become distracted by thoughts, emotions, and other events. We'll now discuss some typical problems tennis players have in controlling and maintaining attentional focus, dividing them into distractions that are internal and those that are external.

Internal Distracters

Some distractions come from within ourselves—our thoughts, worries, and concerns. These irrelevant thoughts can cause players to lose concentration and develop an inappropriate focus of attention. We'll now take a closer look at those *internal distracters* that present attentional problems.

Attending to Past Events

In working with tennis players over the years, this is one of the most often seen problems. That is, players often cannot forget about what just happened on a previous point, game or set—especially a bad mistake that was costly. Focusing on past events has been the downfall of many talented tennis players, as looking backward prevents them from focusing on the present. Here's a comment from a tennis player I worked with who had a problem letting go of past events.

> It was 5-4, 30-40 and my opponent was serving for the first set (but I had a break point). I set up the point well and came to net to put away an easy volley (my opponent was out of court). But I tried to be too cute and I clipped the top of the net and the ball rolled back on my side. I could not believe it. I should have broken him right there. I totally lost it and he went on to hold serve and win the set. I was still fuming when we began the second set and wasn't concentrating at all. I proceeded to be broken in the first game. We remained on serve the rest of the set but I lost 6-4. All because of one missed shot.

Being able to put negative events behind you and wipe them from your consciousness is a critical psychological skill for tennis players. A player needs a narrow-external focus, rather than a broad-internal focus, at this point in time. I will elaborate on this later in this chapter.

Attending to Future Events

Concentration problems can also involve attending to future events. In essence, players engage in a form of "fortune telling" worrying or thinking about the outcome of the event rather than what they need to do to be successful. Such thinking takes the form of "what if" statements, especially prevalent in junior tennis players. Examples include:

- What if I lose (win) this game?
- What if I lose (win) the first set?
- What if I lose (win) the match?
- What if I double fault?
- What if I don't close out the match?

This kind of future-oriented thinking and worry negatively affects concentration, since worrying about what might happen acts purely as a distraction, which can also cause muscle tension and tentative play. For example, Pete Sampras was leading 7-6, 6-4, and serving at 5-2 in the 1994 Australian Open finals. He double-faulted and lost two more games playing tentatively, before holding out 6-4 in the third set. Interviewed afterward, Sampras explained that his lapse in concentration was caused by speculating about the future. *I was thinking about winning the Australian Open and what a great achievement it would be...looking ahead and just taking it for granted, instead of taking it point by point.*

Sometimes the future-oriented thinking has little or nothing at all to do with the particular match or opponent, as your mind can wander without excuse. For example, tennis players report thinking during the heat of competition about such things as what they need to do at school the next day, what they planned for that evening, boyfriends and girlfriends, or going shopping. These thoughts are often involuntary—suddenly players just find themselves thinking about things having nothing to do with the match. This can be very frustrating and makes it all that more important to stay in the present, keeping an external-narrow focus on the ball during points and an internal-narrow focus between points to control your thoughts and emotions.

Choking Under Pressure

Emotional factors such as the pressure of a competitive match, often play a critical role in creating internal sources of distraction. One of these distracters is known as choking, which typically describes an athlete's poor performance under pressure. Tennis great John McEnroe (in Goffi, 1984, pp.61-62) underscores the point that choking is part of competition.

When it comes to choking, the bottom line is that everyone does it. The question isn't whether you choke or not, but how—when you choke—you are going to handle it. Choking is a big part of every sport, and part of being a champion is being able to cope with it better than everyone else.

Although there is little agreement among tennis players and coaches on the exact definition of choking, the general consensus is that it usually results in impaired performance. For example, is double-faulting at match point (down 4-5 in the third set) considered choking? What if you were up 5-4 in the third set and double faulted twice to lose that game but came back to break your opponent's serve and hold your own serve to win the match. Is this a choke? Or did you choke if you won the first set 6-2 and were serving for the match at 5-3 in the second set, had your serve broken and you went on to lose the match. Maybe most interesting is what if you were serving for the match 5-4 in the third set at both 30-30 and 40-30 and you hit very weak second serves but your opponent was overzealous and hit both of them long, giving you the match. Did you choke?

If your responses are anything like those I get from tennis coaches and players in my workshops, then there will not be a whole lot of agreement concerning which situations constitute choking. This is because there are no right and wrong answers, since choking is much more than actual behavior. In fact, it is a process and the player himself or herself is often the only person who can really tell if choking occurred. So double-faulting at match point may or may not be the result of choking. More importantly, we must understand why the player doubled-faulted. In essence, we have to take a closer look at the process that is characteristic of what we have come to call choking.

Behaviorally, we infer that choking has typically occurred when performance deteriorates, especially under situations of high pressure or importance, such as a club championship, a Grand Slam tournament match, a league finals, collegiate championship tennis match, or playing in nationals, regionals or sectionals as a junior. For example, Jana Novotna was serving at 4-1, 40-15 in the third set at the 1993 Wimbledon finals against Steffi Graf and was thus one point away from a seemingly insurmountable 5-1 lead. But she proceeded to miss an easy volley, later served three consecutive double faults, and hit some wild shots, allowing Graf to come back and win 6-4. Wimbledon is considered by many to be the most prestigious tournament to win, and thus the pressure on Novotna was extremely high (note that Novotna did finally win Wimbledon several years later helping to get "the monkey off her back").

In any case, the increased sense of pressure causes you to tighten your muscles. Your heart rate and breathing rate start to increase. The key breakdown, however, occurs at the attentional level. Instead of focusing externally on the ball and opponent, your attention becomes narrow and internal as you start to focus on your own fears of losing and failing. At the same time, the increased pressure reduces the flexibility in your attentional focus, and you have problems changing your focus as the situation dictates. This inappropriate attentional focus coupled with excess anxiety, causes a variety of performance problems such as impaired timing and coordination, fatigue, muscle tension, rushing shots, and poor judgment and decision-making. Thus, the double fault, unforced error, poor choice of shots, missed overhead, or blown volley are simply the end result of inappropriate attentional focus brought about by excess pressure. The choking process is seen in Table 8.2.

Table 8.2	The Process of Choking

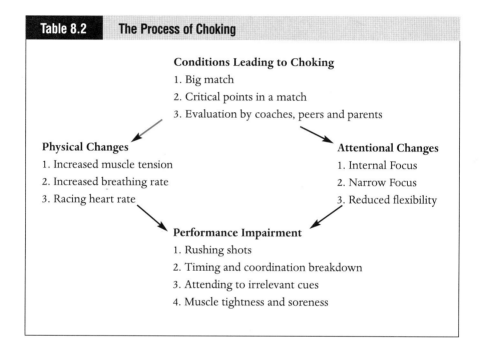

Conditions Leading to Choking
1. Big match
2. Critical points in a match
3. Evaluation by coaches, peers and parents

Physical Changes
1. Increased muscle tension
2. Increased breathing rate
3. Racing heart rate

Attentional Changes
1. Internal Focus
2. Narrow Focus
3. Reduced flexibility

Performance Impairment
1. Rushing shots
2. Timing and coordination breakdown
3. Attending to irrelevant cues
4. Muscle tightness and soreness

Overanalyzing Body Mechanics

Another type of inappropriate attention is focusing too much on body mechanics and movements. This usually occurs when your attentional focus is internal and thus it's important to understand when an internal focus is appropriate. Along these lines, when you are learning a new skill or honing down a skill such as serving, you should focus internally to get the kinesthetic feel of the movement. Using the serve, you might want to focus on the transfer of weight, the scratch-your-back position with the racquet, and the height of your ball toss (although optimally you would focus on only one thing at a time). As you attempt to integrate this new movement pattern, your performance is likely to be uneven. But this is what practice is all about—focusing on improving your technique by getting a better feel of the movement.

The problem arises when internal-narrow thinking continues after you have learned the skill. At this point the skill should be virtually automatic, and your attention should be primarily on what you're doing. So when you are serving in a match, you should not be thinking of all the body mechanics we just mentioned, as this will produce poor performance. But if you start missing and double-faulting, unfortunately, this is what many tennis players start to do. They start to focus on whether they are transferring their weight properly, or if their ball toss is in the right spot, or if they are extending their arm on the follow-through. Although these are all important aspects of the serve, it is not appropriate to focus on these during a match. This overanalysis and internal focus simply produces a *"paralysis by overanalysis."*

This does not mean that no thinking occurs once a skill is well learned. But an emphasis on technique and body mechanics during a match is usually detrimental to performance because the mind gets in the way of the body. The more you analyze, the more likely you are to break the natural, smooth movements, characteristic of high levels of performance. A narrow-external focus on the ball with a minimum of attention paid to body mechanics during rallies will maximize your chances of a good performance. Between points and during changeovers might be more appropriate times to focus internally. Even here, your instructions to yourself must be short and consist of maybe a key word or cue such as *reach, forward,* or *bend.* During the course of a point, however, where rapid decisions and reactions are paramount, an internal focus on your stroke mechanics will likely overload the system, resulting in more errors. During practice is the time to get the feel of the shot and focus on error correction, whereas match play should involve a predominantly narrow-external focus of attention.

External Distracters

External distracters can be defined as stimuli from the environment that divert people's attention from the relevant cues relating to their performance. Unfortunately, for tennis players, a variety of potential distracters exist.

Visual Distracters

One of the difficult aspects of remaining focused throughout a match is that there are many *visual distracters* in the environment competing for your attention. Spectators can cause a visual distraction, which can result in a couple of problems for tennis players. One of the problems arises when you know some of the people in the audience, causing you to start thinking about who is in the audience. Because it is natural to want to look good in front of your friends and family, you may want to impress them with your shot-making ability. This can result in sometimes going for shots that are beyond your ability. For example, you might try to hit a backhand topspin crosscourt winner on the dead run instead of flipping up a more conservative and less spectacular defensive lob. It certainly feels great to hit spectacular shots in front of your friends, but if you try a shot five times and only hit one winner, you are not going to win many tennis matches. In fact, research on "The Championship Choke"

(Baumeister & Steinhilber, 1984) has found that increased self-consciousness placed on athletes by home crowds can cause them to focus too much on the process of movement, causing a decrease in performance.

Besides spectators, many players report being distracted by things going on around them on other courts. I can personally vouch for this distracter as in most tournament situations, we do not get to play on isolated courts where there is nothing else going on. So there is a match typically on either side of you and it is easy to become visually distracted, as you look over to see what's happening on these adjacent courts. I often am tempted to look at the other players (sometimes they are my teammates if it is a team match) to see how we're doing or to check out a possible future opponent.

Auditory Distracters

Most tennis matches take place in environments where various types of noise may act as a distracter to your focus. Common auditory distracters include airplanes flying overhead (typically at the US Open in New York), announcements on the public address system, mobile telephones/beepers, and loud conversations among spectators. Sometimes noises in the form of grunting from your opponent can be distracting, Earlier in her career, several top players complained that Monica Seles' grunting hurt their concentration. As Seles tried to eliminate or at least reduce her grunting, she noted that it impaired her own concentration since she was now not hitting the ball automatically; rather she was thinking about not grunting!

It is interesting to note that auditory sounds and distractions are part of most team sports though very quiet environments are expected for most individual sports such as golf and tennis. Thus, a loud sound from a crowd is typically more disturbing to a tennis player, than it is to a basketball player. I always wondered how a tennis player would serve the ball if there were loud noises coming from the crowd. After all, basketball players shoot free throws with loud noises and hands waving, yet tennis players are totally thrown off if there are some sounds from the audience. That may be one reason why Davis Cup matches are so unpredictable, as visiting players typically never had to play under such loud noise and adverse conditions. One of the reasons that Jim Courier was so successful in Davis Cup, was his ability to go into "hostile environments" and keep his concentration on the match. Maybe practicing with some of these sounds occurring would be helpful in being prepared to deal with them, if they should occur during a competitive match.

Tips for Improving Concentration On-Site

As has been discussed previously, being able to maintain a focus on relevant environmental cues is critical for effective performance. Now it's time to describe exactly how to improve your concentration. Along these lines, I will focus on things you can do on the court. Then I'll suggest exercises that can be practiced at other times and in other places. But please remember that other chapters contain important information regarding how to enhance concentration levels such as the use of imagery (Chapter 7), controlling arousal levels (Chapter 6), setting performance and process goals (Chapter 4), and building confidence (Chapter 5).

Concentration Log

One of the things I typically have the tennis players I work with do regarding concentration, is to enhance their awareness of their level of concentration in practice and matches. Increasing awareness is the first step to making positive changes and is a form of self-monitoring, which is discussed in more detail later in the chapter. This simply means keeping a daily concentration log for practices and matches, recording your thoughts about your concentration that particular day, and any situations that enhance or detract from your concentration (see Table 8.3).

Table 8.3	Concentration Log	
	Date	Observations
Practice / Match		
Practice / Match		
Practice / Match		
Practice / Match		
Practice / Match		
Practice / Match		
Practice / Match		
Practice / Match		
Practice / Match		

Use Simulations in Practice

As noted earlier, there are numerous factors that are often present in match situations that are not normally present in practice situations. Crowd noises, presence of lines people, environmental conditions (sun, wind, temperature), and behavior of opponents, are just some of the things you might come up against in a match that is not normally part of your training environment. All these represent potential distracters and may undermine performance. In research with Olympic athletes, Gould and colleagues (Gould, Eklund & Jackson, 1992; Gould et al.,1999) have consistently found that preparing for unusual events was a prime discriminator between athletes who performed better than expected (won a medal but weren't expected to do so) and athletes who performed worse than expected (expected to win a medal but didn't do so). So what you need to do is prepare for these situations and have strategies set in place to cope with them if they arise during a match. In essence, you try and make practice as close to competition as possible.

Many team sport athletes already train with distractions present such as basketball coaches pumping in crowd noises or football coaches running variations of the two-minute drill. In the same fashion, tennis players should practice with people standing around and talking or with a crowd watching. In addition, if you have trouble playing in the wind or sun, make it a point to practice under these conditions. Unfortunately, many tennis players avoid situations they find aversive. For example, most tennis players hate playing in the wind and thus avoid this situation in practice. But what happens when you have to play on a windy day? The more you practice under adverse conditions, the better prepared you will be to cope with these conditions during matches. Even visualizing playing under these circumstances is helpful. Here's an example of how Jimmy Connors blocked out heat and humidity during a match to maintain his focus:

It was hot out there—really hot—but I knew that if I started thinking too much about the sun, I wouldn't do my best. I didn't worry about it while I was on the court, but when I was sitting down, with the sun bearing down, it started to get to me a little. So I just blocked it out and pretended it wasn't there. That's what you have to do in tennis—not let yourself think about anything that can have a negative effect on your game.

(Tarshis, 1977, p. 45)

Use Cue Words

Put simply, cue words are used to trigger a particular response and are really a form of self-talk (discussed in Chapter 9). They can, therefore, be instructional (*follow-through, watch the ball, stretch, bend knees*) or motivational/emotional (e.g., *hang in there, get tough, relax, stay strong*). The key is to keep the cue word(s) simple and let it automatically trigger the desired response. In hitting the volley, you might use the trigger *firm* or *punch* to emphasize hitting out in front of you with a short stroke. Similarly, in hitting a return of serve, you might use the cue word *forward* to get you moving forward, especially if you have been caught flat-footed before.

To use a personal example, I sometimes had trouble on my second serve hitting out, as I had a tendency to just "bloop" the ball in without taking a full swing. So now, especially on important second serves where pressure is high, I use the cue *reach* before I hit my serve. What *reach* does for me is it emphasizes that I reach up with the ball tossing hand. If I do this, I start to arch my back and it triggers my normal service motion, which almost forces me to hit out on the serve. So cue words need to be meaningful to each particular player. When I consult with players, I have them try to generate a cue word that is meaningful to them, as I find this works better than for me to try to give them a cue. In addition, if you feel that you are not concentrating on a certain aspect of your game, then a cue word might be appropriate in this situation, as shown by Rod Laver's comment regarding footwork and movement.

> *If I can get my feet moving, then everything falls into place a little better for me. Usually when a player isn't concentrating well, it will show up in one or two technical areas, like not watching the ball or not getting the shoulders turned. So rather than simply telling your-self to concentrate, the thing to do is to focus on that one thing that's giving you trouble.*
> (Tarshis, 1977, p. 48)

Employ Nonjudgmental Thinking

One of the biggest obstacles tennis players face in maintaining concentration is the tendency to evaluate performance and classify it as good or bad. Such judgments tend to elicit personal, ego-involved reactions. Judging a couple of shots as bad, for example, will typically result in judgmental thoughts such as "I'm just a choke artist," "I suck," or "I can't play this game." In turn, as noted many years ago by Tim Gallwey (1974) in his groundbreaking book *The Inner Game of Tennis,* these types of thoughts will inevitably make you lose your timing, fluidity of strokes, and rhythm. In essence, your brain starts to override your body, causing excess muscle tension, excess effort, concentration lapses, and impaired decision-making.

Instead of judging the worth of your performance and categorizing it as either good or bad, you should learn to look at your actions non-judgmentally. This does not mean that you should ignore errors and mistakes; rather you should simply see your performance for what it is, without adding judgments. For example, let's say that you have missed almost all of your passing shots into the net. This does not mean labeling your passing shots as terrible, which usually leads to anger, frustration, and disappointment. Your observation that most of the shots went into the net provides information that possibly you are turning your wrist over too fast. In response, you try to keep your wrist a little firmer on passing shots in an attempt to improve the situation. Thus, in this way, the player has used his performance evaluation constructively, which translates into better performance and a more enjoyable experience.

Establish Routines

Routines can focus concentration and help mentally prepare for an upcoming performance. Researchers have argued that pre-performance routines work by helping players divert their attention from task-irrelevant thoughts to task-relevant thoughts. In essence, routines increase the likelihood that players will not be distracted internally or externally, prior to and during performance. This often allows the performance to stay automatic, without interference of conscious awareness. In addition to a pre-performance routine, breaks in the action are ideal times for routines, as the mind likes to wander during these times. For example, a tennis player during changeovers might sit in a chair, take a deep breath, and image what she wants to do in the upcoming game. Then she might repeat two or three cue words to help her focus attention before taking the court. In this way, time is structured during this "dead time" and used to keep the player in the match, focused, and planning what to do next. Two of the major areas where routines can be helpful for tennis players during play, are the serve and service return. The serve is the only stroke in tennis completely under your control. In addition, you either start all points with a serve or service return. So you have a little time to plan on what you would like to do. Top players have planned, practiced, and perfected their routines so that they can feel comfortable throughout a match. A good routine reduces anxiety and focuses concentration on the critical aspects of the serve and service return. Table 8.4 contains suggestions for both serve and return of serve routines. However, these, as other routines, need to be individualized to meet your specific needs, abilities, and preferences. We will discuss the use of routines to prepare for a match in more detail in Chapter 10.

Table 8.4	Serve and Service Return Routines

Serve Routine
1. Determine Positioning and Foot Placement
2. Decide on Service Type and Placement
3. Adjust Racquet Grip and Ball
4. Take a Deep Breath
5. Bounce the Ball for Rhythm
6. See and Feel the Perfect Serve
7. Focus on Ball Toss and Serve to Programmed Spot

Service Return Routine
1. Decide on Where and How to Return Serve
2. Take a Deep Breath and Take Your Ready Position
3. Picture the Desired Service Return
4. Focus on the Server and Ball Toss
5. Use Cue Words

Develop Competition Plans

In-depth interviews with elite athletes in a variety of sports clearly indicate the importance of establishing pre-competition and competition plans, to help maintain their attentional focus (Greenleaf, et. al., 2001). These plans help athletes not only prepare for their events, but also prepare for what they would do in different circumstances, both before and during competition. In most cases, athletes design these detailed plans of action to facilitate attentional focus on the process of performance (as opposed to factors over which they have no direct control, such as the actions of other competitors and final outcome).

This notion of planning is certainly applicable to tennis players, as they prepare for a specific opponent or match. The key thing from a concentration point of view is to make sure you know what you generally want to do, but that you are also prepared for different circumstances and possibilities. In this way, your concentration stays focused on the match regardless of how the match unfolds. This comment from a collegiate tennis player captures this idea:

> I would always have some sort of plan for an upcoming match. I would go over it with my coach if possible and it would be as specific as I could make it. The more I knew about an opponent the more specific it would be. This helped me maintain my concentration throughout a match, since I was always focused on doing a specific thing. Even if things went wrong, I was prepared for that also.

Stay Present-Focused

In Chapter 2, we discussed the importance of staying in the present as one of the keys to achieving peak performance. Of course this is easier said than done, as the mind likes to wander away from the point at hand. But great players have a unique ability to stay focused on the present, ignoring the past and future. As an old saying goes, "you can't do anything about the past but you can ruin a perfectly good present by thinking about it." All time great Bjorn Born was once asked what he felt was his most outstanding attribute, helping him be one of the greatest players of all time. Borg, who certainly was gifted physically with quickness, stamina, and timing, commented as follows: *It was my ability to play one point at a time and not worry or think about what just happened or what might happen. The only thing that was important was the point about to be played* (Phillips, 1980, p. 56).

The interesting thing is that Borg learned this skill, as he was known to have temper tantrums on the court and lose his cool when things did not go his way. In fact, it got so bad that his parents put his racquet in a closet and forbid him to play tennis for 6 months. So he needed to learn to play one point at a time and not let things bother him if he was going to play at all! Throughout this chapter and Chapter 9, I will provide you with techniques and strategies to help keep you focused in the present, such as thought stopping, and changing self-talk.

Self-Monitoring

Research by Kirschenbaum and his colleagues (see Kirschenbaum 1997 for a review) has clearly indicated that simply *self-monitoring* can enhance concentration and improve performance. But what exactly is self-monitoring? All you are really doing when you self-monitor is observing yourself in a systematic fashion. In essence, if you want to change a behavior, you would observe that behavior on a regular basis. The observation might include writing down when the behavior occurs, or simply recording under what conditions the behavior is displayed. Self-monitoring typically improves behavior because it makes your goals clear and important. Self-monitoring essentially puts a mirror in front of you as you perform. This "mirror," shows you how you are doing compared to your goals, thereby encouraging you to work harder to reach those goals. Research has revealed that the number of elements practiced by figure skaters increased by 67% for those who self-monitored (Hume, Martin, Gonzalez, Krackley & Genthon, 1985). In addition, they decreased from 8 minutes to 2 minutes the amount of time spent off-task (e.g., talking to others, taking breaks, standing around) in a 45-minute session.

Applying this to tennis, you could simply self-monitor the time spent (or number of attempts) practicing a given shot such as the overhead, serve, approach shot, or volley. The point would be that the mere fact of self-monitoring would increase your focus on that particular shot, since we know that we tend to shy away from practicing things on which we need the most work. The more repetitions you were able to achieve in practice the better that particular shot will usually get in matches. Table 8.5 provides you with a sample self-monitoring form you could use during practices to help you get a better feel for how often, or under what circumstances, you were practicing different strokes or strategies.

For example, you might simply practice your backhand cross court hitting many repetitions as your coach feeds you balls. This might take 10 minutes. However, you might also play a game where you have to hit your backhand cross court against a partner and you keep score up to say 15 points (you lose a point when you don't hit the ball cross court). This might also take 10 minutes but the circumstances have changed. You or your coach could also create specific game situations and then play out backhand cross court points. Or maybe you simply want to get some match experience and play sets against a teammate. In any case you would be monitoring the amount of time spent working on different things such as stroke production or competitive play. I have always been amazed at the lack of focus in practice as many players simply just hit ground strokes back and forth without any real purpose. Self-monitoring should help focus the practice and provide you with feedback as to exactly what you are doing on the court during practice. This might surprise you but should also help you focus on what needs to be done during practice.

A variation of self-monitoring that has been proven to be effective in enhancing athletes' performance is known as *positive self-monitoring*. In this case, you would basically do the same thing as outlined above except you would pay attention to, and note only the positive aspects of a given stroke or strategy. For example, let's say you were working on improving your serve and you did this for 15 minutes during practice. You also created certain game situations so that the serve might simulate more actual match conditions. In positive self-monitoring, you would also note the positive aspects of your practice serving (you do not focus on the negative at all). In this case you might have recalled that your ball toss was just the right height and out in front of you to provide you with more power. You might also recall that you went through your pre-service routine before each serve. Finally, you also noted that you really got your racquet back in the *"scratch the back"* position which added speed to your serve. Kirschenbaum (1997) noted that this positive self-monitoring (a) helps you remain focused on the task at hand, (b) improves confidence, (c) decreases negative emotions, and (d) reinforces persistence. Self-monitoring and positive self-monitoring take a little extra time, but the results in improving your game will be exceptional.

Table 8.5	Self-Monitoring of Practice	
Strokes/Strategies	**Time on Task**	**Situations Created**
Forehand		
Forehand down-the-line		
Forehand cross court		
Backhand		
Backhand down-the-line		
Backhand cross court		
Forehand volley		
Forehand volley cross court		
Forehand volley down-the-line		
Backhand volley		
Backhand volley cross court		
Backhand volley down-the-line		
Forehand approach shot		
Backhand approach shot		
Overhead		
Serve		
Groundstrokes - Short Angles		
Groundstrokes—Depth		
Doubles		

Overlearn Skills

As I have noted several times throughout the book, your mind has to be freed up to let your body work at maximum efficiency. In Chapter 2, the importance of performing on "automatic pilot" was emphasized as it related to peak performance. In essence, to perform at high levels, athletes report that *overlearning* of the skills involved in their sport helped concentration in the competitive environment. In interviews, athletes consistently stated that the skill they were required to perform in competition had to be overlearned to the extent that they could stay focused, despite any distractions that might be present (Hardy, Jones, & Gould, 1996). Overlearning frees up one's attention to concentrate on other aspects of the performance environment and helps make the performance of the skill automatic.

For a tennis player, this would mean executing strokes and patterns of play over and over again in practice, so that you don't have to think much about them during a match. One thing overlearning does, is allow you to perform more than one task at a time, which is important to a tennis player. Most shots in tennis have to be accomplished very quickly and there is not a lot of time to think about how to hit the shot, what shot to hit, as well as your opponent's court positioning and tendencies, the score of the game or set, etc. So overlearning allows you to make these complicated decisions quickly because you do not have to exert much attentional processes to actually hitting the ball (since you should be able to do this on automatic pilot based on overlearning the skill), which leaves attention left over for making these decisions.

Practice Eye Control

Like the mind, the eyes tend to wander away from the task to irrelevant cues and distractions, such as people in the crowd, players playing on the next court, antics of your opponent, or planes overhead. *Eye control* can help keep your eyes focused on the relevant cues in your own match, such as the ball and opponent. Several players I have worked with darted their eyes around the court and outside the court and ultimately they became distracted by what they saw. One good way to keep your eyes from wandering is to focus them on a single object like the strings in your racquet. Thus, between points, keeping focused on your strings will effectively prevent you from looking around and focusing on other irrelevant cues. It doesn't have to be your racquet strings, but the key is to pick something that can maintain your focus of attention and prevent your eyes from picking up distractions. This is what one professional player did to keep his eyes focused throughout a match.

> It starts when you walk out on the court. I always tried to simply look down at the ground or my feet, especially between points and games. I never looked up at my opponent (except during actual points), umpire or anybody else. I did not listen to any voices that might be coming from the crowd or elsewhere. I simply kept my eyes focused on the court and my opponent during points and just kept my head down between points and games. That's how I kept my concentration throughout a match.

Exercises to Improve Concentration

Besides the various things you can do during a match to help focus your concentration, there are a couple of specific drills you can work on during practice sessions to improve your attentional focus.

Different Colored Balls

This exercise can be accomplished by use of a ball machine or someone feeding from a basket of balls. Fill the ball machine (or basket) with balls of two colors (e.g., white and yellow) and place the machine on the opposite baseline. Designate one color ball as *down the line* and the other color as *cross court*. It is then your job to watch the ball closely, determine its color, and then hit the ball down the line or cross the court. This will force you to really focus on the ball so you can determine its color early and then perform the appropriate response. To increase difficulty, simply move the ball machine closer to the service line which puts increased emphasis on watching the ball and picking up its color early. If you don't have different colored balls, the person feeding the balls can simply call out a "1" (down the line) or "2" (cross court) as the ball is hit. Balls can be hit quicker or the feeder can move toward the service line to increase difficulty.

Thought Freezing

Since concentration wanders so frequently, it is important to develop a mechanism for examining the contents of your focus in practice. Arrange a tennis drill in which you determine beforehand what kind of focus is necessary for optimal performance. For example, when practicing forehand cross courts, a narrow-external focus on the path of the ball is required to execute the skills. Next, have your partner shout out the word "freeze" at various unexpected points throughout the drill. At exactly the moment you hear the word "freeze," stop what you are doing and quickly describe the contents of your focus to your partner. This exercise will put you more in touch with your affect, thoughts, and kinesthetic feelings. So you would not only be getting feedback about the attentional focus needed to perform this task, but also your own attentional focus at that point in time. The exercise is a lot of fun and challenges your partner too. You can shout out "freeze" to her also as she performs different skills, so both parties will benefit in different ways.

Consecutive Groundstrokes

This drill is designed to improve concentration, patience, and discipline (all important in winning tennis matches). Depending on your skill level, choose a specific number of ground strokes that you would like to hit without making a mistake (e.g., 10, 20, 30, 40). Have someone feed you balls or hit against a ball machine and try to reach your goal. If you miss you have to go back to zero and pressure increases as you approach your goal (because you don't want to start all over again at zero). You can increase the difficulty by requiring that the ball land in a particular part of the court (e.g., past the service line if you are working on depth, or cross court or down the line). You can also do this with other shots like volleys and overheads; the possibilities are limitless and the end result will be more focused concentration and mental discipline.

Fast Exchange

This drill will help you learn to keep your mind in the present moment and not wander. Use a ball machine that has a fair range of velocities. Stand at the net in volley position and then have someone set the machine at a comfortable speed. Gradually increase the velocity, and you should see that you become more and more concentrated. As balls come at you very quickly, you must pay full attention or else get hit on the side of the head. There is no time to let the mind wander. You should try and stay calm and relaxed and totally focused on the ball in the present.

Decision-Making

As noted earlier, you have to literally make hundreds of decisions throughout a tennis match. Constantly having to make decisions is stressful and one of the reason most players hate to play good "pushers." Specifically, you never know when is a good time to approach the net, so you are constantly debating with yourself whether you should approach or not. This exercise takes some of the decisions away and actually forces you to make certain decisions. Draw a line approximately three feet behind the service line on your side of the court (the distance could vary depending on your own particular needs and abilities). Whenever your partner's shot lands between this line and the net, you must approach the net. This means moving toward the ball early, maybe before it bounces, so that you can take it early and on the rise if possible. Your partner then has the option of either hitting a passing shot or a lob.

CHAPTER 9

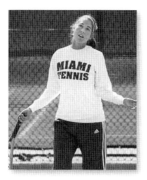

SELF-TALK

The previous chapter focused on the concept of attentional focus, including definitions, types, problems and ways to improve. This chapter is closely related to the concept of proper attentional focus in that *self-talk* can be seen as simply another internal distracter. But self-talk plays a huge role in tennis performance and deserves to be addressed in a separate chapter. In fact in working with tennis players over the years developing mental skills, I probably do more work with the concept of self-talk than any other mental skill. So I will focus on understanding the nature of self-talk, how it relates to performance, common problems with self-talk, and ways to make self-talk work in our favor. Let's start defining what we mean by self-talk and discussing the different types of self-talk.

Types of Self-Talk

All of us who play tennis talk to ourselves with some degree of regularity. Of course, the frequency and content will vary from individual to individual and from situation to situation. Self-talk can be a distracter, but it can also be a way to deal with distractions. When sport psychologists refer to self-talk, they typically refer to it as thinking or making internal or external statements to yourself. Although we typically think of self-talk as being internal to the person, it can also be external and heard by others. Of course we hear lots of self-talk on the tennis court (imagine what we are not hearing) so it's instructive to understand what it does to a player's affect, thinking, and performance. So first, let's try to classify self-talk.

Positive and Negative Self-Talk

One of the traditional ways in which self-talk has been categorized is whether it has positive content (*positive self-talk*) or negative content (*negative self-talk*). Positive self-talk is typically seen as an asset that enhances self-esteem, motivation, attentional focus, and performance. By using a specific set of positive verbal cues, tennis players can keep their minds appropriately focused on task-relevant cues. Positive self-talk also helps you focus on the present and keeps your mind from wandering. More recently, this positive self-talk has been broken down into *motivational* and *instructional* self talk.

Motivational self-talk typically has to deal with athletes trying to keep themselves up for competition and keeping their "heads" in the competition (especially when it is long term and very difficult) when they might be losing or behind. Some examples might include, *"hang in there," "get tough," "I can do it,"* and *"stay focused."* In motivational self-talk, there is no specific information on how to perform the skill or persist; rather it simply tries to keep you pumped up and into the competition. Conversely, instructional self-talk provides specific information on how to perform the skill more effectively such as *"keep your eye on the ball," "bend your knees," "keep your wrist back,"* and *"firm wrist."* Depending on the situation, motivational or instructional self-talk might be more appropriate. Recent research (Theodorakis, Weinberg, Natsis, Douma, & Kazakas, 2000) has revealed that instructional self-talk appears more appropriate and effective when dealing with a complex skill such as tennis (unless you are tired and need some motivation to keep trying and persisting).

Finally, it is interesting to note that recent research (Hardy, Gammage, & Hall, 2001) has demonstrated that self-talk usually comes in one of three categories including single cue words (e.g., *"breathe," "relax," "concentrate"*), phrases (e.g., *"come on," "move forward," "get tough"*) and short sentences (e.g., *"Don't worry about past mistakes, focus on the ball," "Keep your wrist firm and eyes on the ball"*). Of the three, phrases was used most often by tennis players as self-talk needs to be short and to the point.

The one type of self-talk I have not discussed so far is known as negative self-talk. Unfortunately, this is the most prevalent of the different types of self-talk, especially in tennis. In fact, in a study of competitive junior tennis players (most of whom held sectional USTA rankings) by Van Raalte, Brewer, Riveria & Petitpas, (1994), it was found that 96% of the players used negative self-talk. Of these players, 88% used negative self-talk at least 13 times in a match (and this was only the self-talk that was actually heard by observers). As might be expected, in almost all cases, negative self-talk followed points that had been lost. Negative self-talk is typically critical, self-demeaning, and anxiety producing, as well as undermining confidence, and reducing concentration. In spite of these potentially negative outcomes, we still hear lots of negative self-talk on the tennis court such as *"you stink," "how can you possibly hit a shot like that," "you're so stupid," "your serve sucks,"* and *"you can't play this game."*

Uses of Self-Talk

Self-talk has a variety of uses that are both psychologically and physically-oriented. I will briefly discuss these uses as they pertain to tennis.

Breaking Bad Habits (or Old Habits)

Most tennis players develop at least one bad habit (usually several) during their playing days and breaking that habit is often difficult. In essence, you have to unlearn an automatic response and learn a new response. So switching from a one-handed to two-handed backhand, or from an Eastern grip to a Western grip, places severe demands on our concentration. Trying to change a learned bad habit such as not getting your racquet back soon enough or pushing your backhand because you get too close to it, also requires lots of effort and concentration.

You (along with your coach or teaching pro—if you have one) should help decide on the most relevant cue or cues that will help make the new response automatic. Therefore, some type of instructional self-statement would appear most appropriate. The greater the change, the more self-instruction will be necessary. Remember to focus on what you want to do such as *"keep your wrist firm"* not what you don't want to do such as *"don't tighten from the elbow."*

Initiating Action

To initiate action on the court, motivational self-talk appears to be best although sometimes instructional cues might also be helpful. For example, if you were feeling lethargic in a match and not moving well, you might use motivational self-talk such as *"move," "quick,"* *"pick it up,"* or *"get going."* If your serve lacked *"pop"* you might use words such as *"explode,"* *"forward,"* or *"reach."*

Skill Acquisition

Learning new skills, whether as a beginner or more advanced player, can benefit from the use of self-talk strategies. However, in either case, make sure the self-talk chosen is short and meaningful to you. This type of self-talk tends to be instructional in nature, as you are trying to cue yourself what to do. As you become more proficient, you will need fewer and fewer cues as your strokes become more automatic. In addition, your cues for a serve, for example, might focus more on where you want your serve to go, than on how to actually hit it.

Sustaining Effort

Just like self-talk can be used to initiate action, it can also be used to keep you motivated and putting forth effort as a long match draws on. Of course you want to be in good physical condition, but positive, motivational self-talk such as *"hang in there," "stay with it,"* and *"keep it up"* can also be useful cues to keep a sustained effort.

Enhancing Psychological States

The main emphasis of this book is on how to develop psychological skills to help improve your tennis performance and your tennis experience. Most certainly, self-talk can help initiate these types of states (although you still have to practice them individually like we discussed earlier in the book). But cue words such as *"relax," "focus,"* and *"confident"* can bring into the forefront these important mental states.

How Self-Talk Works

We are not disturbed by things, but rather the view we take of them.

Epictitus

There is nothing either good or bad, but thinking makes it so.

Shakespeare

The above quotes highlight the importance that our thoughts play on how we evaluate and respond to events in our life. It is typical for most people to feel that some things are good (e.g., getting married, winning a match) while other things are bad (e.g., getting a divorce, losing a match). But in reality, events are simply events. It is our evaluation of events that make them positive or negative and this in turn determines our emotional and physical responses to the events.

For example, you might have recently broken up with your girlfriend (boyfriend) and feel that this is terrible and awful. You feel depressed, frustrated, and really down. However, someone else in your same situation is in much better spirits, much more upbeat, and optimistic. So here is the same exact situation, but people are reacting very differently. Events are the same but people's reactions to them are very different, due to their perception and evaluation of the event.

Let's take a tennis example. You are playing in the finals of an important tournament and you are up 4-1 in the third set (two service breaks). However, you start to tighten up and think ahead to winning the championship. As a result you play more tentatively and your concentration is compromised. On the other hand, your opponent starts to hit out more and actually starts hitting winners and you wind up losing 7-6 in a tiebreaker. You can't believe you lost the match and are depressed, mad, and frustrated about blowing a 4-1 lead in the third set. In fact, this really "takes the wind out of your sail," and you lose motivation to continue to work hard because you just can't seem to win the big one. Now consider the same scenario except that you change your self-talk and perspective after the match. Specifically, instead of getting mad and upset, you say to yourself, *I really wanted to win, but the match showed me that I have to work a little harder in practice on staying calm and focused as I try to close out a match.* So you realize you have the ability to win and are motivated in practice to work harder to try and put everything together.

This illustration highlights the idea that events, in and of themselves, do not cause your emotional reactions such as depression, anger, hopelessness, frustration, calm, and optimism. Rather, it is how you interpret an event that really determines your response. This relationship between an event and response, mediated by your perception and evaluation of the event (self-talk) is presented in Table 9.1. As can be seen in the table, your self-talk plays a crucial role in not only how you react to an event, but also your future feelings and actions as noted above. Note the differences in reactions when the same event is perceived differently, and your self-talk is different.

Table 9.1	Process of Self-Talk	
Event (Environmental Stimulation)	**Self-Talk** (Perception/Evaluation)	**Response** (Emotional, Behavioral Physiological)
Unhealthy Examples		
Losing an important match	I can never win the big one	Discouragement, depression, frustration
Missing an important shot during a tennis match	You're an idiot—you can't win playing like this	Anger, hopelessness muscle tension
Healthy Examples		
Losing an important match	I know what I need to do in practice	Optimism, motivation calm, concentration
Missing an important shot during a tennis match	Just relax—there's plenty of tennis still left	Relaxation, optimism, focus

Self-Talk and Performance Enhancement

Although both practitioners and researchers have argued the potentially important benefits of positive (motivational and instructional) self-talk in enhancing task performance, it has only been in the last 5-10 years that empirical research has corroborated this assumption. One of the studies noted earlier focusing on tennis, was conducted by Van Raalte et al (1994). They investigated audible self-talk in junior players (so they missed everything players said to themselves) but still found some interesting results highlighted below:

- Losers used more negative self-talk than winners and this negative self-talk was usually evidenced after a mistake.
- Winners and losers did not differ in the use of positive or instructional self-talk.
- Players who believed that their self-talk influenced the outcome of the match won significantly more points than did non-believers.

- 96% of the players used negative self-talk at least once and 88% used it at least 13 times (compared to 21% who used positive or instructional self-talk 13 or more times).
- 55% of the players used positive self-talk (mostly motivational).

Other studies, as well as our own research, have consistently demonstrated the effectiveness of positive and instructional, self-talk specifically on tennis performance. Instructional self-talk appears best when you are trying to learn a new skill during practice or recovering from a mistake during the match. The self-talk, should act as a way to get you to focus on a specific aspect of a stroke or remember to do a specific thing (e.g., *bend your knees, short backswing*). When you're trying to get or stay pumped up, motivational self-talk appears to be best as this non-specific talk (e.g., *hang in there, get tough*) acts to get the body going and keeps you focused and motivated in practices and matches. So if certain types of self-talk are so good for you, then your first step would be increasing your awareness of the types of self-talk you employ, and when you employ them.

Increasing Awareness of Self-Talk

Unfortunately, most of us are not really in touch with our self-talk, and thus we can't alter what we don't know. Therefore, carefully reviewing the way in which you use self-talk can help you identify beneficial and detrimental kinds of self-talk, and the circumstances or match situations bringing out different kinds of self-talk. One way to get a better understanding of the relationship between self-talk and your tennis performance is through retrospection, coming either right after a match (which is really a form of self-monitoring), or reflecting on your best and worst performances.

Retrospection/Self-Monitoring

One good time to identify and understand your self-talk is right after a match (or practice). Specifically, as soon as possible after a match, make a list of your thoughts and self-statements, situations in which they occurred, and performance consequences. In essence, try to recall your thoughts and verbal reactions to a variety of situations throughout the match. If possible, have someone videotape a tough match with close-ups of your facial expressions and verbalizations. This will further help you identify self-talk in various situations (of course you'll still have to identify what you were saying to yourself at different times since this would obviously not get on the tape). In monitoring your self-talk, pay particularly close attention to the types of situations and events that trigger negative self destructive, self-talk which undermine your performance (see Table 9.2). These might include: (a) losing your serve, (b) missing an easy shot, (c) losing a big point, (d) double-faulting, (e) blowing a lead, and (f) making an unforced error.

Another form of self-monitoring which I have used successfully with tennis players is to have them start a match with a bunch (50 or so) of paper clips in their right pants pocket. Every time the player would make a negative statement, I would have the player put a paper clip into his left pocket. In one particular case, at the end of the match, the player was amazed at how many paper clips were in his left pocket. He said to me, *I knew I was negative sometimes but 38 paper clips in my left pocket was really a wake-up call that I was really getting down on myself.* This exercise could be followed up by writing down the situations in which you were negative, to see if there was any pattern to the negative statements.

In addition, it is also instructive to try to remember your best and worst recent performances. As you do this, attempt to identify and record the content and frequency of your self-talk. Most tennis players can identify their self-talk and usually notice a distinct difference between these two situations. Specifically, good performances are usually characterized by positive and instructional self-talk, whereas negative performances are usually accompanied by negative self-talk. These two types of retrospection should help you to get a better handle on the situations that produce negative self-talk (as well as positive self-talk), which is the first step to making your self-talk more productive.

Table 9.2	Identifying Your Self-Talk

Positive Self-Talk　　　　　　　　　**Situation**

_____

_____

_____

_____

_____

_____

_____

Negative Self-Talk　　　　　　　　　**Situation**

_____

_____

_____

_____

_____

_____

Techniques to Improve Self-Talk

To this point, I have tried to define what self-talk is, its uses, its different types, its effects on performance, and how to become more aware of it. So now it is time to learn and develop some techniques and strategies to enhance the quality of your self-talk.

Thought Stopping

One "tried and true" method of coping with negative statements is to try to stop them before they really enter your consciousness and undermine your performance. The technique of *thought stopping* is designed to stop these negative thoughts before they become harmful and is borrowed from clinical psychology (originally developed to deal with obsessive thoughts).

Thought stopping begins by training yourself to stop whatever you were doing, when you hear the word "STOP." The word "STOP" acts as a cue or trigger to stop paying attention to the undesired thought and refocus your attention. This reduces the probability of letting negative events carry forward to the next point or game. Of course you can use other cues to stop paying attention to undesired thoughts, such as snapping your fingers or hitting your hand against your thigh. Choose whatever works for you.

Although it sounds easy, thought stopping is difficult because it involves not only being aware of your thought process on the court, but also breaking a bad habit of negative self-talk that you might have been doing for a long time. Many people believe that breaking bad habits involving the way we think should be easy. But this is far from the case. You know how long and how many repetitions it takes to break a bad physical habit such as taking your racquet back too high on your backswing, or getting too close to the ball when hitting a backhand. In fact, in my consulting with young tennis players, I have found that they often have 20-30-40 negative thoughts in a given match, so trying to stop each one of those thoughts is a difficult proposition. So don't expect total success to come right away.

To get better at stopping our thoughts, again takes practice, and we should start using this technique on the practice courts. In the first step, whenever you start thinking a negative thought (and of course are aware of it) just say "stop" out loud (or whatever cue you use) and then refocus on a task-relevant cue (such as the ball or possibly your racquet strings between points). You should have a cue ready and available to you so that when you stop focusing on the unwanted thought, you should immediately turn your focus to a more task-relevant cue. The point of saying "stop" out loud is to indicate to you and your coach (or tennis teacher) that you are working on your new skill. After you start to master saying "stop" out loud, then you can start saying it to yourself. Moving from an external cue to command stop to an internalized one such as thinking stop in your head, may take some time to accomplish. If you are having trouble concentrating after one particular situation (such as missing an easy shot), then you might only focus your new technique on this situation. As you overcome this problem and start to feel more comfortable with the "stop" technique, you can move on to other troublesome areas.

Another way to practice stopping unwanted thoughts is through the use of imagery discussed in Chapter 7. This has the advantage of practicing thought stopping without actually being out on the court. Using this approach, you would attempt to visualize (using all appropriate senses) a situation in which you have had trouble with negative statements. Visualize this situation as vividly as possible including the negative statement you would typically use. You would then use your stop cue to interrupt these thoughts. In working with tennis players, I have found it to be especially helpful to actually visualize a red stop sign in your head as this really highlights the need to stop.

Changing Negative Self-Talk to Positive Self-Talk

In the best of worlds, it would be best to totally eliminate negative self-talk, but this is not entirely realistic, as negative thoughts have a way of entering our mind. So the next best thing is to change these negative thoughts into positive ones and direct your attention back to the task at hand. In Table 9.2, I asked you to keep track of your negative statements and the situations under which they were made. Once these negative statements have been recognized, then your job is to replace these negative statements with positive ones. Table 9.3 provides an illustration of some typical negative statements made by tennis players and some possible positive replacement statements. The key thing is to use statements that make sense to you and can effectively counter the negative statements that may undermine your performance and compromise your enjoyment. Like thought stopping, you should use it in practice (as well as in your imagery) before attempting it in a match. Since negative statements happen more often under stress, in a match, try to stop the negative self-talk and take a deep breath. As you exhale, try to relax and repeat the appropriate positive statement.

Countering Irrational Beliefs

At the core of much of the negative-self-talk we see on a tennis court, is an underlying belief in these statements. World-renowned psychotherapist, Albert Ellis (1962), has termed these beliefs irrational beliefs. In essence, these beliefs or thinking are counterproductive since they can undermine your confidence, motivation, self-esteem, enjoyment, and performance. Although there are many irrational beliefs, in my work with tennis players, these are the ones that appear most often, and are most destructive. I also provide some suggestions for countering these irrational beliefs.

- *My performance on the court reflects my worth as a person.* This is one of the most debilitating and destructive of all the irrational beliefs. You feel great when you play well and win, but are down in the dumps when you play poorly and lose. You have the feeling that friends and family members will like you more when you win, but will think less of you when you lose. In essence, you perceive that your self-worth is on the line whenever you play competitive tennis. However, you should separate your self-esteem from your performance on the court—people who matter will not change their opinion of you based on your performance on the tennis court.

Table 9.3	Changing Negative to Positive Self Talk	

Negative Self-Talk	(change to)	Positive Self-Talk
You stink		It's just one shot –hang in there
I never play well in the wind		It's windy on both sides of the court. Just play the wind
I hope I don't choke again		Relax and just watch the ball
How could you hit such a stupid shot		Just focus on the next point
Your serve is the worst		Just go through your routine and slow down a bit
What if I lose this match?		Just enjoy playing. Winning and losing will take care of itself
That was the worst line call I ever saw		I can't control line calls. Just play your game
I can't believe I missed that shot		Everyone makes mistakes—just focus on the next point
I'll never win this match		Just play one point at a time

- *I should be able to play perfect tennis.* This type of belief only leads to frustration and disappointment. But with all the negative self-talk one hears on the court, you'd think lots of players expect to make every shot (but even the pros miss easy shots). Nobody plays perfect tennis, and believing that you can, only increases your muscle tension, creates unrealistic expectations, leading to poorer performance. A more realistic view would be to accept the fact that you will make mistakes but will learn from these mistakes.

- *Playing poorly early in a match means playing poorly later.* Unfortunately, this is a belief held by many young tennis players and will often lead to giving up or not putting forth consistent effort throughout a match. In this way you simply confirm that you were having a bad day from start to finish. Research and experience have clearly revealed, however, that you can never accurately predict later performance from earlier performance. Sometimes you start off playing poorly, but by the end of the match are playing great (and vice versa). Therefore, you need to believe in yourself and expect to play better as the match progresses, even if you got off to a slower start than usual.

- *Being critical of myself helps my performance on the court.* Research from a variety of sources, indicate that criticism (especially constant) is detrimental to performance. Even John McEnroe has gone on record saying that being critical and losing his cool hurt (rather than helped) his performance and game. Instead of being self-critical (e.g., *You're an idiot—you can't play this game*) it is much more productive to be self-evaluative and provide yourself with instructional cues to correct and enhance your behavior (e.g., remember, a short backswing on your volleys).

- *I can't learn anything from losing a match.* This probably relates to the emphasis that society has placed on winning. So after losing a match, many players simply pout, become upset and just try to forget about it. But you can learn a great deal from losing, especially if you can take some of things you did not do well and work on those in practice. But also remember what you did well, as this might be important to a game plan for future matches.

CHAPTER 10

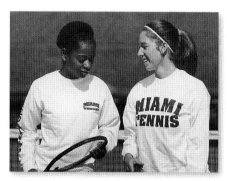

MENTAL PREPARATION

My feeling about preparing for a match was always this: that I wanted to do as much as I could ahead of time to prevent distractions. I was a creature of routine. It was always important for my peace of mind to have gotten a good night's sleep the night before, to have eaten at the right time....I was finicky about my equipment. I always had to make sure my racquets were strung right, and that I'd gone out and warmed up enough to get a feel for the sun, the wind, and the bounce. ... I found that if I didn't make sure of all these things ahead of time I'd start to think about them a little bit during the match and it affected my concentration

Jack Kramer
(Tarshis, 1977, p. 37)

One of the first lessons I learned when I turned pro in 1982 was how much of an edge could be gained before the match even got started. It became obvious to me that for the best players in the world, their match had begun a long time before the first serve. They came ready to play and wanted to grab me by the throat as soon as they could.

Brad Gilbert

The above quotes by all-time great Jack Kramer and tennis pro, coach and author, Brad Gilbert illustrate the importance of preparing yourself to play competitive tennis. In the previous chapters, I have focused on developing mental skills in practice and at home to help maximize your tennis game. These all come together in getting yourself ready to play a competitive match. You probably remember times when you had to race to the court from school or work or that something important was on your mind, and thus your mind was not really focused on the match. In essence, you simply lacked the time to mentally prepare. This probably resulted in less than optimal performance. The focus of this chapter will be to provide a structure for effective mental (and physical) preparation and help you avoid some of the common pitfalls of poor preparation. Of course, each player will likely need to develop his or her own pre-match preparation, but these general guidelines should help you develop your own unique approach.

Pre-match Preparation

There are different aspects to getting mentally and physically prepared for an upcoming competitive match. One of the things that you can do before actually getting ready to play (both mentally and physically) is to develop a solid game plan, so let's address this issue first.

Developing a Game Plan

As Allen Fox (1993, p. 125), tennis author and former top 10 player has said, *Before playing the first point of a match, it is absolutely necessary to have in mind a game plan—a basic set of strategic guidelines for your play.* Unfortunately, game plans that establish a strategy of how to play a specific opponent, are often overlooked by tennis players. The game plan, in essence, gives your efforts structure and provides direction, without which you are like a cross-country driver without a map. Without a game plan, you just hit shots back, and do not really decide on how best to play a specific opponent. Your pre-match planning in a sense creates a mental compass. You know where you want to go and how to get there. There may be detours along the way and your opponent may present some surprises, but the basic route is laid out in your head in advance and your mental compass keeps you on course.

To formulate a game plan requires that you analyze and list your opponent's mental and physical strengths and weaknesses, matching these against your own strengths and weaknesses. This task is obviously easier if you have played against your opponent before (which is usually the case in competitive tennis), but it also can be done by observing players or even gathering information from other players who have played this particular player. Some particular questions you might ask yourself in assessing an opponent's game (in this case assuming you have played this person before) include the following:

(a) Who won most baseline rallies?
(b) Were you successful in coming to net?
(c) How was your opponent's volley?
(d) How were your opponent's first and second serve?
(e) How did your opponent handle lobs?
(f) Did your opponent serve and volley? (which serves?)
(g) Did your opponent attack your second serve?
(h) Did your opponent prefer to pass cross-court or down-the-line?
(i) Did your opponent "fight" the entire match?
(j) How did your opponent play crucial points (aggressively, conservatively)?

After assessing your opponent, it's time to realistically assess yourself. Many tennis players, unfortunately, don't always realistically assess their capabilities. Rather, just because you are capable of hitting a shot, does not mean you can consistently hit it or hit it under pressure. So even though you aced your opponent eight times last match and got in 65% of first serves, you normally only get in 45% of your first serves and only occasionally hit an ace. Therefore, you wouldn't want to depend on a big first serve as a part of your game plan. More to the point, the key is that you match up your strengths with your opponent's weaknesses. In addition, consider how to protect your weaknesses from being exploited by your opponent's strengths (see Table 10.1, which provides an example of how a game plan is devised and executed).

Table 10.1	An Example of a Game Plan and Its Execution

Brad Gilbert provides a good example of developing a game plan against Boris Becker in preparation for their US Open. He notes the following things after carefully observing and examining Becker's game:

(1) Becker like to attack my second serve.
(2) Becker loves to hit with great pace.
(3) Becker sometimes can get frustrated if you keep him on the court a while.
(4) Becker has a great forehand, but is more inconsistent on that side.
(5) Becker will hit some unbelievable shots.
(6) Becker likes to pass on his backhand down the line.

In looking at the strengths and weakness in his own game, Gilbert devised the following plan to compete with Becker (Gilbert knew that his physical game could not match up to Becker's physical game and presence). So his game plan for Becker was:

(1) Increase my first serve percentage so that Becker has fewer chance to attack my weaker second serve.
(2) Try to create some mistakes on his forehand side by hitting soft with little pace.
(3) Don't be impressed with anything he does. Let him hit great shots but make him hit them over and over. Always try to make him hit one more shot.
(4) Put forth total effort on every point. Try to extend the match and keep Becker on the court for as long as possible.
(5) Serve to his forehand regularly. Look for a short crosscourt return and come to net and look for the down-the-line passing shot.

As it turns out, Gilbert's game plan highlighted in Table 10.1 worked exceptionally well. He was patient and although he lost the first two sets, he seized an opening in the 3rd set (after being behind 3-0) and kept on executing his game plan to perfection. Becker started missing forehands, and he got more and more frustrated as he played longer and longer. Gilbert eventually won in 5 sets.

Once you decide upon your game plan you should make a commitment to carry it out to the best of your ability. However, a game plan is a funny animal. On the one hand you need to commit your full mental energies to its execution, but you need not be so rigid, that you cannot change or adjust it if necessary. Even if you know nothing about your opponent, you should still construct a game plan based on your own strengths and weaknesses and carry it out until your opponent's actions tell you to change.

So the tricky part of your game plan is that although you need to be fully committed to it, you also need to be evaluating its effectiveness throughout the match. If you're winning easily and playing well then there is usually no problem. But it's when you're losing and starting to feel out of control that you need to start considering changing your game plan. The great champion, Bill Tilden is credited with coining the old adage, *Always change a losing game plan; never change a winning one.* Of course this makes perfect sense but the difficulty comes in determining if your game plan is working or not. If you are losing 6-1, 5-1, it's usually too late to change your game plan. But my experience has been that players have a tendency to give up on game plans too soon. For example, if part of your plan is to come in on short balls, making your opponent hit backhand passing shots (because you feel this is a weakness), and you get passed twice in a row, you might come to the conclusion that this was not a good plan and stay back and trade baseline shots. But this would probably be jumping to conclusions too quickly since two passing shots does not a match make. While your opponent may be able to hit a couple of passing shots early in the first set, can he do it at 4-5 30-30 for example, when the pressure is on, or can he do it consistently throughout a match? If you give up too early, you may never find out. Also, when some players leave a game plan too early, they are not really sure what game plan to use to take the place of the original one, since they only came prepared with one plan. This usually results in players getting panicky and emotional which oftentimes leads to a poorer choice of shots and eventually poorer performance.

Let us assume for a moment that your initial game plan is a losing one. What kind of change should you make? First of all, it would be helpful if you come prepared with an alternative plan as this keeps attention focused and confidence high. The key point about any new plan (or original plan for that matter) is that it is within your capabilities. This may seem obvious but it is often lost in the emotions you are experiencing at the moment. Let me give you an example from my own playing experience. I was playing in the finals of a tournament against an opponent who was known to be very steady, making you win points because of his rare unforced errors. In the first game of the match, not only did I play steady, but I took short balls and hit them either for winners or placed them deep in the court for easy volleys on the next weak return. I won that game without losing a point. Then my opponent started serving the next game, and amazed me by serving and volleying. I had never seen him do this in his previous matches and in fact he did not have a particularly good serve or volley (but he did have very consistent ground strokes). I went on to win that game easy and won the match in a lopsided 6-0, 6-0.

After the match my opponent said, "After the first game I knew I couldn't hit with you so my only chance was to serve and volley." My opponent made two classic mistakes regarding changing his game plan. First, he changed his game plan too soon. Just because I played a good game, my opponent assumed I was not going to miss any shots, thus I did not have the opportunity to go for and miss big shots on important points (which I have been known to do on occasion). The second error my opponent made was changing his game in a manner that emphasized the weaker, not the stronger, part of his game. There was no way he was going to beat me serving and volleying, because he simply was not that good at it. In essence, he went away from his strength—consistent ground strokes—to focus on a game plan that was not within his capabilities. So by changing his game plan he really decreased his chances of winning instead of increasing them.

So what could my opponent have done, given that his initial game plan wasn't working. Well since his strength was consistent ground strokes, he could have stayed with his strength and attempted to keep his shots deeper and the points going longer. This would have kept me from hitting winners on short balls and increased the chances that I would make a mistake trying to over hit. Would this new game plan have worked? I certainly don't know (and am glad he didn't try it) but I do know that this would have been playing more from his strength rather than simply giving up the baseline strategy. Although I don't know if it was the case in this particular situation, in general, when players adopt strategies that are outside their capabilities, it is often their own way of covertly quitting. The key points in setting up a good game plan are highlighted in Table 10.2.

Routines

In Chapter 8, we briefly discussed the concept of routines in terms of increasing a player's concentration. Although routines are certainly important during a match, they are also important as part of your pre-match mental and physical preparation. In general, routines should do two specific things: (a) help organize your time so you can progressively focus on the match, and (b) remove uncertainly from your environment. If you don't prepare yourself to play a match, then you leave yourself open for distractions from a mental perspective, or are not ready to play physically. NCAA champion Allen Fox (1979, p.72), noted earlier, relates the following story about how his lack of mental preparation made him unprepared to play a match.

I was due to play Jon Douglas in the Pennsylvania Grasscourt Championship. I had beaten him twice before already that year on concrete and now we were going to play on grass which was Douglas' worst surface. I thought the match was a lock so I got myself involved in a two-hour chess game right beforehand. So I brutalized my mind through a two-hour marathon and, when I got to the court to play Douglas I felt physically weak. Worse than that, I found that I was so emotionally drained that I did not have the mental strength to concentrate for the length of time it would take to win the match. Inevitably, I lost. I had gone out there poorly prepared and had paid the price. Bad preparation begets bad results.

Table 10.2	Key Points to Setting Up and Changing a Game Plan

Setting Up A Game Plan

(1) Gain a clear understanding of your own and your opponent's strengths and weaknesses.

(2) Decide on a general plan of how to win most of the points.

(3) Are you going to be better off with offense (hit winners) or defense (retrieve and wait for your opponent to make an error).

(4) Decide specifically on how to carry out your general game plan (e.g., in general, you want to take the offensive and become more aggressive. Specifically, you decide to come in to the net on second serves and balls that hit inside the baseline and approach to your opponent's backhand side).

Changing A Game Plan

(5) Change your game plan because you optimistically hope your new plan will be better than your old one, not because you simply want to "throw in the towel."

(6) Make sure the new game plan is within your capabilities. Just because you have done something occasionally does not mean that you can do it consistently.

(7) Pursue your new game plan with all the will, energy, and commitment you can.

The previous example highlights the importance of getting yourself physically and mentally prepared for a match. Getting ready involves a variety of physical and mental actions that prepare you for maximal performance as you get closer and closer to match time. These might include formulating a good game plan, being at the right emotional level, being focused on the match, getting the proper rest, eating the right foods at the right times, stretching and warming up. This preparation might seem like a lot but it's essential if you are to play to the best of your ability.

Besides getting you ready to play, the other reason for having a consistent pre-match routine is to remove uncertainty from your environment. Earlier in Chapter 5, we noted that lack of control was one of the most important stressors for athletes. Of course there are many things a tennis player can't control (e.g., the sun, wind, playing surface, antics of opponents) but one of the things totally under your control is what you do prior to playing. Sometimes these actions (e.g., warming-up, stretching, imagery) have specific functions; but other times they are simply part of your routine and might border on superstitious behavior.

What these types of behaviors do, is to provide structure and consistency to your pre-match preparation. Tennis players most certainly have their fair share of superstitious behaviors, which do serve an important function so they should not be minimized. In working with many players and playing tennis myself for many years, I have come across many of these superstitious behaviors involved in pre-match preparation. These include things such as wearing certain "lucky" shorts or shirts for a match, always putting on the right (or left) shoe and sock on first, making sure your last warm-up serve was not a fault, wearing a wristwatch when you play, and always starting on one side of the court (north or south) regardless of playing conditions. What all these disparate behaviors have in common is that tennis players associate these actions with successful performance, despite the fact that how you play should not depend on which shoe you happen to put on first. But that is precisely the meaning of superstition—the misapplication of cause and effect. Somehow we have come to believe that certain shirts will cause us to play better and it is this belief that is so important. If you believe putting on your right sock will help you play better, then it probably will (see Chapter 6 on confidence and the self-fulfilling prophesy). The key point of all of this is that you should develop a routine that you are comfortable with and that you can depend on, regardless of the situation. Some of this preparation might be purely based on what makes you feel good, whereas other parts should work specifically on doing certain things, physically and mentally, to get you ready to play your best. When you walk out onto the court you want to feel that you have an edge; this usually helps your confidence and performance.

Although routines are really important and helpful, there are times when you will be unable to carry out your routine due to circumstances beyond your control such as a flat tire, family crisis, business meeting, or school commitment. Therefore, you need to be flexible enough to alter your preparation and still play at a high level. So if your routine is broken, you need to still be able to play well and thus not become over dependent on your routine. You might develop a back-up or alternative routine that you can do so at least you maintain some control in preparation for a match. I will now provide you with some general suggestions regarding different areas that might fit into your pre-match routine. Choose those aspects that are good for you and devise your own pre-match routine that is individualized and comfortable for your style, personality, schedule, and ability. You can use Table 10.3 to write out the different aspects that go into making up your routine.

Sleeping/Rest

Of course, to consistently play your best, you need to get the proper amount of rest and sleep. So on a day-to-day basis you want to be well rested averaging eight or more hours of sleep per night. In terms of pre-match preparation, sleep sometimes becomes a problem since players often have difficulty getting a good night's sleep prior to an important match. But overall, moderate amounts of sleep deprivation produce relatively few problems with sport performance. Here are a couple of pointers regarding getting a good night's sleep prior to a match.

- Use any of the relaxation techniques discussed in Chapter 6.
- Alcohol can increase tiredness; however it causes awakenings later in the night and should be avoided as a way to enhance sleep.

- Avoid caffeine 4-6 hours before bedtime.
- Avoid vigorous exercise 2-3 hours prior to bedtime but regular exercise earlier in the day may improve the quality of sleep.
- Try to go to sleep at a set regular time.
- Avoid heavy meals 2-3 hours before bedtime.
- Minimize excessive noise, light, heat, or cold during the sleep period.

Table 10.3	Setting Up Your Individualized Routine

Game Plan

Rest (Sleeping)

Eating

Equipment Check

Stretching

Mental Preparation

Warm - Up

Equipment

Although it may seem like a small point, as part of your pre-match routine, it's a good idea to check to make sure you have everything you need in your tennis bag for playing and for injury. Brad Gilbert (1993), in his book entitled *Winning Ugly*, recommends the following be brought to the court in your tennis bag. Although some of this might seem a bit much, you never know what might go wrong so it doesn't hurt to be prepared. The list includes (a) water, (b) two or more racquets, (c) tape/band aids, (d) energy food, (e) ibuprofen, (f) grips, (g) cap with a visor, (h) towels, (i) sweatbands, (j) dry shirts, and (k) chemical ice. You never know what might happen on a given day so why not be prepared.

Eating/Drinking

Food is a critical element to a player's pre-match routine, as mistakes in food/drink intake can really make a difference in performance. In fact, there is now a multi-million dollar industry out there catering to athletes' and coaches' views of the foods and drinks that supposedly make people perform better. Unfortunately, many of these views distort reality, so it's important to have up-to-date scientific evidence regarding food and drink effects on performance. Many of today's top players adhere to a relatively balanced diet; there is no "one size fits all" when it comes to when and what to eat. So I will provide some general guidelines to follow to maximize performance in developing your general eating/drinking patterns as well as eating/drinking in relation to your pre-match routine (see Eisenman, Johnson, & Benson, 1990, *Coaches Guide to Nutrition and Weight Control* for a more detailed discussion).

But a point to follow is to generally adhere to a balanced diet that represents the five different food groups. The American Dietetic Association recommends (a) 6-11 servings per day from the grain group (e.g., breads, pasta, cereal), (b) 2-4 servings from the fruit group, (c) 3-5 servings from the vegetable group, (d) 2-3 servings from the milk group (e.g., milk, yogurt, cheese), (e) 2-3 servings from the meat group (e.g., meat, poultry, fish, eggs), and, (f) sparing use of fats, oils, and sweets.

- *Eat a balanced, high carbohydrate, low-fat diet.* Research has revealed that consistently eating a diet that is high in carbohydrates (50% or more) such as potatoes, pasta, cereal, bread, and rice and low in fat (less than 20%) is most beneficial to performance. If you avoid eating anything fried, red meat, regular cheese, anything cooked in oil, and typical dessert items (e.g., cakes, pies, cookies, ice-cream), you can get your diet quite low in fat.
- *Protein and vitamin supplements are usually not necessary.* In looking at the diets of athletes, it has been found that they typically eat sufficient amounts of proteins and do not need protein supplements. Foods such as milk (including skim), chicken, yogurt, no-fat fish and turkey and other high protein foods should be included in your diet, but it need not account for more than about 20% of your daily caloric intake.

- *Pre-competition meal essentials.* This meal should consist of foods that are easily digested, easily absorbed and focus on complex carbohydrates totaling about 300-500 calories. About 2-3 hours before the match is optimal to maximize energy and provide sufficient digestion time. A few pre-meal suggestions are listed below.

  (a) Two corn muffins, one tablespoon of jam, one cup of skim milk, and one-half banana.

  (b) One english muffin, one tablespoon of jelly, one cup of non-fat fruit yogurt, one cup of orange juice.

  (c) One cup of corn flakes, one cup of skim milk, one cup of orange juice. A liquid meal could be taken one-hour before competition (although more time is still recommended) since they empty the stomach quickly. These meals should not be high in sugar content but should have some protein and carbohydrate in them.

- *Drinking.* Drinking fluids regularly as well as in preparation for a match is very important, especially if you are playing outside on a hot day. In day-to-day use, you should drink several glasses of water per day (not tea or coffee or soft drinks since they contain caffeine). You should start drinking water a couple of hours before the start of a match so the body gets a head start on absorbing them into the system. We tend to drink when we're thirsty and dehydrated (during a hot match) which is good, but we should be drinking even if we are not thirsty. So drink after the first changeover, even if you're not thirsty. Don't wait until your tongue is hanging out to start to drink; get started early and keep drinking.

Stretching

Many tennis players now do a lot of weight lifting and cardiovascular training to get them in top shape to play competitive tennis. This is a good practice, but players often underestimate the importance of daily stretching as part of one's pre-match routine. Unfortunately, many top players have been temporarily or permanently sidelined with a host of injuries, since tennis is a very demanding game. There are three primary benefits from stretching and they include:

- *Reduce the probability of injury.* Injuries play a big part in tennis careers and being able to stay away from major injuries is in part luck but also preparation and training. Several top professional players had careers end early due to persistent injuries, while others have struggled and not reached their potential due to injuries. There are a host of tennis-related injuries such as tennis elbow, shoulder problems (rotator cuff), heel spurs, back problems, stress fractures, and knee problems. Many of these originate in the teenage years when players are putting in many hours to develop and hone their skills. One of the things that you can do to prevent injury is to stretch on a regular basis, but also make it part of your pre-match routine. By increasing your range of motion due to deliberate and slow stretching, you also reduce the probability of injury.

- *Increase performance.* By increasing your flexibility, you are also benefiting performance because you can generate more power through a fuller range of motion. For example, as you take your racquet back to serve, it is important that your muscles are supple and relaxed, so you can lay your racquet way back by extending your arm behind your head.
- *Relaxation.* Stretching has also been shown to relieve excess tension, which is related to increases in performance (see Chapter 5). In addition, focusing your mind on the muscles being stretched can serve the purpose of eliminating anxiety-producing thoughts concerning the upcoming match.

There are a variety of books that provide detailed information regarding proper stretching, along with a host of specific stretching activities for different parts of the body. Therefore, I will provide only a few guidelines and suggestions regarding stretching as part of your pre-match routine, as well as some general points about stretching.

(a) Spend about 10-15 minutes on pre-match stretching exercises.

(b) Perform all stretches gently and slowly, stretching to the point of tension and holding the stretch for a minimum of 10 seconds. Each stretch should be done three times. Since stretching is best accomplished when muscles are warm, try to increase circulation prior to stretching. So, for example, if you like to hit prior to your official warm-up, after the hit would be a good time to stretch (as is after the match when muscles are very warm).

(c) Focus on the muscle groups that might give you (or have given you) trouble. Although you want to include all major muscle groups, be sure to include the back, hamstring, shoulder, forearm, and calf areas as these are most prone to tennis injury.

(d) Do not bounce when you stretch. You want static (slow and controlled) stretching.

(e) If you are on a team, one of your teammates might help with some stretches.

(f) When you stretch out a muscle, exhale as this increases relaxation and enhances flexibility.

Imagery

If you have gotten sufficient rest, eaten properly, and stretched, you are getting your body ready to play. But of course, you need to get your mind ready to play and a great way to do this is through the use of imagery. In Chapter 7 we discussed the use of imagery in detail, so I won't repeat it here. However, as you get yourself mentally ready to play, you want to accomplish several things including: (a) focus your thoughts on the match; (b) achieve your optimal level of arousal; (c) build up your confidence; (d) get the feel of your shots; and (e) review your game plan. Imagery can help you achieve these thoughts and feelings.

You (possibly with your coach or teaching pro) can devise an imagery script in preparation for a match (a generic imagery script is provided in Chapter 7). In the script should be several components that will accomplish the different aspects noted above. For example, you want to see yourself hitting smooth, efficient ground strokes, crisp volleys, and getting the rhythm on your serve and return of serve. This will help not only the feeling for your strokes, but also build confidence and a positive attitude. In your imagery you should also see yourself playing out points that reinforce your game plan. If you want to attack your opponent's weak second serve, then see yourself stepping up in to the court and hitting safe but aggressive returns and following them with put away volleys. Your imagery should also help focus your mind on the match and help reduce or eliminate irrelevant, anxiety-producing thoughts. Remember to use the principles of imagery discussed in Chapter 7.

Warm-Up

The last part of your pre-match routine and preparation should be your warm-up. Most recreational players waste or minimize this part of the pre-match routine because they don't understand how much it can contribute to winning. The warm-up is your final opportunity to set the stage for getting off to a good start; to get a jump on your opponent that can affect the entire match. There are basically five things that you want to accomplish in your warm-up:

(a) Continue to loosen-up and warm-up the body which was started via your pre-match routine;

(b) Work on your timing while settling down and reducing tension;

(c) Familiarize yourself with environmental conditions/court surface;

(d) Increase your confidence; and

(e) Learn as much as you can about your opponent.

As you start your warm-up, you should hit your ground strokes deep, just inside the baseline. This helps program the body for hitting deep in the match and works against tension, which tends to shorten shots. Now you should add some spin including topspin and slice and you might even try a specialty shot like a drop shot to help get the feel and range. Work on your weaker side as well as your stronger side—now is not the time to run around shots. Remember, you are not trying to impress your opponent with your speed and power; rather you are just trying to develop a rhythm and get some timing on your shots.

Now you want to step in the court a bit and hit a couple of balls on the rise and then eventually hitting an approach shot off a short ball. Hit your first volley by the service line and then move in toward the net for your second volley, followed by volleys from both sides. Then warm up your overhead smash just trying to make good contact; don't worry about angles or power. Now you are ready to take some serves and make sure that you serve to both the deuce and ad courts as well as hit your first and second serve. You'll need all these serves once the match starts so you might as well practice them. Just try to get a good rhythm going and slowly add pace and accuracy to your serves. Finally, make sure you get in some service returns as you get a feel for your opponent's pace, direction, speed, and spin of serve. Your timing here is important and this can be started during warm-ups. This should all lead to you feeling more confident and comfortable with your strokes.

While you are warming yourself up, you should also be studying your opponent's game, picking up strengths, weaknesses, and any little pieces of information that you might use in a match (e.g., he likes to take a big looping swing on his forehand side). Some of this information might include: Is the person right or left-handed? Does the person hit with slice or top-spin? How well does the person move? How are his or her first and second serves? Remember not to be impressed with anything your opponent does in practice because oftentimes this does not resemble what happens during a match. This information should be incorporated into your game plan (discussed earlier) or maybe if you know your opponent well, it already has been. In any case, you want to be clear about what your opponent does well, and does not do well, because you want to make your opponent hit shots that are uncomfortable as often as possible.

Finally, you should be carefully analyzing and getting familiar with the particular environment conditions and court surface. Understanding the speed of the court is crucial along with how different spins react, distance behind the baseline, lighting, background, and any other peculiarities. If playing outside, the wind and sun become important factors to consider. Different strategies and shot selection may be necessary depending on which way the wind is blowing, or if the sun is behind or in front of you.

CHAPTER 11

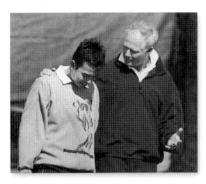

PSYCHOLOGY OF MATCH PLAY

Throughout this book I have discussed different mental strategies and techniques (e.g., imagery, anxiety management, goal-setting, routines, self-talk, etc.) that could be used to enhance your performance and enjoyment in tennis, including those that can be employed in preparation for a match. I have emphasized that tennis is a lot more than the ability to hit certain shots, along with speed, strength, and endurance (although these attributes are certainly important). Rather, it is oftentimes a mental struggle (above and beyond one's physical talents and abilities). In essence, you have to be able to recognize and take advantage of opportunities and understand what's going on during a match. This involves using both the left and right sides of your brain. The right side lets you perform at high levels and is spontaneous and creative. This is the side that's most likely working when you are performing up to your potential. Tim Gallwey (1974), in his groundbreaking book, *The Inner Game of Tennis*, focused on this right side which is more intuitive, and free of analytical thought. But you also need your left side to analyze and interpret situations and then make some calculated decisions on what shots to try and where to try and hit them. Brad Gilbert (1993), in *Winning Ugly*, focused more on the left side of the brain where the goal is to outthink your opponent. In this chapter of the book, I will try to incorporate both perspectives in providing common examples of how to use (and sometimes combat) psychology throughout a competitive tennis match. Remember, the player with prettier, more grooved strokes does not necessarily win the match. It is the winner of the mental game that usually is victorious (and has more fun).

Mind Games

A good way to get started is to look at the following quote by all time great Bill Tilden, who definitely recognizes the importance of the mental side of tennis:

I would rather destroy my opponent's confidence by forcing him into an error than by winning outright myself. Nothing destroys a man's confidence, breaks up his game, and ruins his fighting spirit, like errors. The more shots he misses, the more he worries, and ultimately, the worse he plays. That is why so many are said to be off their game against me. I set out deliberately to put them off their game.

(Tarshis, 1977, p. 119)

Tilden was very perceptive in realizing that errors really gnaw at a player and slowly erode his or her confidence. This is one very subtle way to get "inside the head" of your opponent and simply might be seen as good strategy (in fact after one of my league matches that I won handily, my opponent said to me "I haven't made this many errors in all my matches combined." I simply thanked him but felt that I almost always made him hit another shot to win the point which led to a lot of his errors, since he went for a lot on many of his shots). But there are lots of mind games that occur within a tennis watch. Oftentimes it is not always easy to tell the difference between good strategy and gamesmanship. The rules of tennis are usually very clear relating to the physical aspects of the game (e.g., height of the net, length of the court, scoring, etc.) but they are not always so clear when it comes to psychological conduct. In essence, what is good strategy to one player seems like bad sportsmanship to another. In either case, you need to effectively deal with the situation, or if you are creating the situation, be sure that it is within the rules of play.

Let's take a couple of situations and see if you think these are examples of good strategy or gamesmanship. You are playing an opponent whom you have played several times before (and you won most of the time) but today she is "in the zone" and can't seem to do anything wrong. In particular, her forehand is really on and she is hitting winning forehands from all over the court. So during a changeover, you casually say, "I can't believe your forehand today, you're really hitting everything right near the line." This certainly seems like an innocent comment and in fact you are complimenting your opponent. But now, your opponent suddenly becomes conscious of her forehand and she really is trying to hit the lines with almost every shot, whereas before she was simply hitting the ball smoothly and instinctively (right brain). Now the ball starts to drift just beyond the lines, as she is paying close attention to her forehand. In essence, your comment acts as a little distraction, which takes your opponent off her game just a bit. Is this an example of good strategy or gamesmanship?

You are playing a good opponent who is playing very well this match. You lose the first set and are down an early break in the second set. You feel the match slipping away from you and you need a break of serve. So you slow things down. You are slow to get back into the ready position to receive serve and then keep your head down picking your strings until you are ready to play (you are not using too much time, rather you are taking the maximum time allotted between points). One rule of tennis is that you play at the pace of the server (who is ready to serve before you are ready to return). But another rule is that the server cannot serve until the receiver is ready to receive serve. So your opponent can't serve while you have your head down and are not ready to receive. Your opponent gets mad at your "slow down" tactics and starts to go off his game. You eventually come back and win the match. Was this good strategy or gamesmanship?

Your answers to the gamesmanship versus good strategy questions are not important. What is important is that you recognize and understand these type of situations (whether you consider them gamesmanship, good strategy, or psyching-out an opponent). There are basically two different types of psyching that can hurt you. The kind that your opponent does to you and the kind that you do to you. But in either case, the end result is typically a disruption in your concentration. These antics, situations, or tactics can upset your emotional equilibrium and tempo, and take you out of your game. Instead of controlling the pace and tempo of a match, you are being controlled. Therefore, the next section will focus on some of these typical mind games as well as how you might effectively cope with them.

Warm-Up-Psych-Outs

A good place to start is in the warm-up because this is a prime time for the use of mental ploys. This is especially the case when you are playing a new opponent, but warm-up ploys can also be used for familiar opponents. This is a time when you are learning more about your opponent and evaluating his or her strengths and weaknesses (in addition to getting the rhythm and timing of your own strokes). Let 's look at some of the areas within the warm-up where your opponent may employ some gamesmanship.

Types of Shots

One thing players can do is not let you warm-up properly. Specifically, they don't hit you the kind of balls you want and thus you can't get your timing down. So, for example, when you come up to hit volleys they decide to work on their passing shots, or when rallying from the baseline, they hit the ball wide and either you let it go or have to run hard to get it (increasing the chance of injury). In essence, you don't feel properly warmed-up and are already mad and upset at your opponent. Another ploy is for your opponent to hit great shots during practice, trying to tear down your confidence. They hit deep, with good pace, hit crisp volleys and boom in their serve (as well as crack their return of serves). But most times, players are unable to hit these types of shots (at least with consistency) in a match, so you need not be too impressed. Frankly, if they could hit these shots consistently they would probably be playing on the professional circuit.

Verbal/Non-Verbal Communication

We communicate both verbally and non-verbally and each of these can provide an avenue for gamesmanship in the warm-ups. Your opponent can say (or do) lots of different things regarding his or your game, weather conditions, court conditions, match importance, or injury status, that can throw off your concentration. Some of these verbal ploys might include:

- Can you hit me some shots with some pace?
- I can't believe the poor lighting on these courts
- I hope my ankle injury doesn't flare up today
- It's so hot out here, I don't know why we even have to play this match
- I hope I have enough energy to play after being out late last night

Similarly, some typical non-verbal ploys used during warm-ups that are aimed at working on your psyche include the following:

- Purposely avoiding any eye contact with you
- Carrying a bunch of high priced racquets
- Dressing in cut-offs and black socks
- Dressing in very expensive tennis clothes

Match Psych-Outs

After you have been on the lookout for warm-ups ploys, now a whole new set of mental games can start once the match is ready to commence. Remember that winning tennis matches is as much a mental struggle as it is a physical struggle. So here are some mental games that people play during matches to get a psychological advantage.

Hooking (Line Calls)

One of the things that distinguishes tennis from other sports and adds to its difficulty, is the need to call your own lines (i.e., no referee) in most situations (besides professionals). The unwritten rule for line calls is that you should give your opponent the benefit of the doubt if you are not sure of a call. But if you clearly see a ball out (even though it was close) then you should call it out. The problem arises when you play against that occasional person who intentionally (or unintentionally) makes bad line calls. Probably nothing gets players so upset and mad as feeling that their opponent is making unfair line calls. Concentration and focus can be lost as can emotional control. It's frustrating because your opponent has the final say on balls that land on his or her side of the court. So what should you do when you perceive that you have gotten a bad call?

First of all you should not argue on a marginal call. Oftentimes you might be wrong and maybe didn't see the ball correctly. I have a little exercise I do with junior tennis players to make the point of the difficulty of calling lines. I stand up about 10 players on the service line and I hit a ball (standing next to the players on the service line) to the opposite baseline. I ask them to immediately signal "in" or "out" when the ball bounces. When I get a ball near the baseline, I usually get several players calling it in and several players calling it out. In this case, all the players had to do was watch the ball and call it in or out (they weren't moving around and playing as they normally would be during a match). The point of all this is to demonstrate how difficult it is to call lines and what we see (or perceive) might be different from our opponent. So, you should let marginal calls go by. You might simply give the place where the ball hit a longer look without saying anything, as this signals to your opponent that at least you weren't sure about the call.

If you really think you got a bad call, then you should simply ask your opponent if she was sure of the call. If your opponent says she is sure, then leave it at that. If you start off by accusing your opponent of making a bad call, she'll probably just get defensive and make more of the same. An early notice that you expect fair calls will often sharpen up your opponent's eyes. If you nudge someone about a call in a subtle way, you'll almost always get the benefit of the doubt on the next call. So being diplomatic is encouraged. If it happens repeatedly, most club players start to make bad calls of their own. This is not advisable ethically since it is wrong and it can also destroy your concentration, since now you're thinking too much about calls and not enough about winning the match. At this point you might ask for a linesman if one is available. This will usually settle the issue.

If there is no tournament referee, then the best thing to do (although not always the easiest) is to put it behind you and continue playing (some of the concentration skills discussed earlier would be helpful). There are but a few tennis matches that are decided by a line call or two. The problem is when one line call affects your subsequent play. The better player usually wins and if you keep your composure and play your game, you will maximize your chances of being successful. Finally, if this is recreational tennis, you can simply cross this player off your list of future opponents. But if it's in a tournament, stand up for your rights but do it without insulting your opponent.

Playing Slow

Earlier in the chapter, I gave the example of a player slowing down the pace and asked if this was good strategy or gamesmanship. If it is within the rules it would probably be good strategy, although if it is done against you (and is effective), you would probably think of it as gamesmanship. The point is, when would it be beneficial to slow down and what do you do if an opponent slows down the game against you? Although somewhat counterintuitive, it is usually the player who is ahead who has more pressure, since that player is expected to win the match and thus expectations are high at this point. If you are behind, it's a good idea to slow things down a bit to let your opponent think a little more and feel the pressure. This could mean walking to pick up a ball far away from you and taking your time either getting ready to serve or return serve. This would make the match more mentally draining for your opponent who simply wants to get off the court with a win. You are taking advantage of the rules rather than stalling or breaking the rules. This might also have the effect of breaking up the flow and rhythm of your opponent.

Another way to slow down a match is simply slow down your pace of shot. Most good players like to hit against some pace as this feeds into their own games. It is more mentally demanding and challenging to play against someone who hits with little pace but keeps the ball high and deep. Players have a tendency to over hit against "moonballs" and often get impatient leading to unforced errors. In fact, many players don't consider this type of playing, real tennis. But remember, good strokes do not win matches; a match is often a battle of wills and minds, not strokes. Along these lines, when one person was asked to describe what I did well on the tennis court, he simply responded "he knows how to win." I took this as a compliment since it really meant that my mental game was strong.

Now, what if you are playing against someone who was playing slow? I remember a match a while back with two great Australians playing against each other on slow clay; John Newcombe and Rod Laver. Newcombe managed to win in three sets although clay was not his favorite surface. He played the match very slowly and deliberately. When asked (in a somewhat critical manner) about his slow style of play after the match by a TV commentator, Newcombe replied, "it must have been a good way to play." So what do you do against such players? The key is to play your game and not get involved in their game if they are simply playing slow (but within the rules). It's their right to play slow (in fact you might want to play slow, so you can think out your strategy and deal with anxiety more effectively), so you just have to accept it and keep focused on what you need to do to win points. If you start getting upset because they are slowing down the pace of the game, then your opponent has gotten inside your head. You need to simply stay with your game plan and keep focused on the present, using appropriate self-statements (see Chapter 9) that are instructional in nature, that keep you focused on the things you need to do to be successful.

If your opponent slows down the pace of shots, you need to remain patient and wait for a short ball with which you can hurt your opponent, Here, patience and discipline are the keys and you need to wait for your opportunities (and there will be opportunities). You might also prepare yourself for such situations by using imagery prior to the match (see Chapter 7). In this way, you could see yourself being patient and disciplined in these types of situations, taking a short ball and aggressively hitting it. This puts your opponent on the defensive and then you can see yourself putting away a volley or overhead. Finally, actually practicing against such strokes in simulated match conditions can also be effective. You can have your coach or playing partner hit you high looping balls and you can practice what to do in these situations. This type of simulated practice could be used to prepare for a variety of mentally trying situations such as (a) playing a match with little warm-up, (b) having play stopped as your opponent argues a line call, (c) playing against an opponent who is constantly yelling at himself, (d) getting a bad line call, (e) playing with lots of noise and people moving about, and (f) playing against an opponent who really slows down the pace of a match or who simply plays slowly.

Opponent Distractions

Another common ploy used by players is to try to distract opponents via some sort of emotional outburst. This might take the form of an emotional outburst on the court, challenging a line call, berating themselves, or bringing the crowd into the match. In most cases, this has little to do with whom they are playing, but the end result is a disruption to their opponents' concentration. Sometimes this is calculated and sometimes it just happens; but in either case you need to deal with it effectively and maintain your concentration.

A prime time to try to distract an opponent is when he or she is gaining control of the match and is feeling confident. So if you are winning a match 6-3, 2-1 (up a service break in the second set) it may be time for your opponent to try to stop this momentum and get back in the match. Sometimes, even a slight break in the action is enough to throw a player off his or her game. So simply questioning a line call and taking some extra time (even if the line call is not reversed) will often be enough to get a player to lose concentration (possibly thinking about the line call in question). Of course, players who try to distract their opponents through their own antics, need to make sure that they don't distract themselves. Although John McEnroe appeared to be the master of this psychological ploy, he sometimes lost his cool during these outbursts costing him important matches (like the French Open against Ivan Lendl in 1984). Once again, instructional, task-relevant self-statements that focus on your game plan would be appropriate, as would imagery that prepared you for such a situation. Just don't get caught up in the antics of your opponent; stay focused on what you need to do to be successful.

Compliments

Especially in recreational tennis, players often compliment opponents on good shots. Tennis players, like other people, like to be complimented and told that they did a good job or gave a good effort. This makes us feel accepted, worthwhile, and competent. But you rarely hear this at the professional level. The reason is that players do not want other players to feel good, confident, and comfortable. You should model this type of behavior from the pros. Specifically, you should avoid acknowledging good shots from your opponent, verbally or non-verbally. After your opponent makes a great shot, just go about your business and walk at your normal pace with your normal expression to start the next point. This tells your opponent that you were not impressed with his or her shot making ability and most certainly are not upset or disturbed by it. By keeping your expression constant and not acknowledging the shot, you show your opponent that you mean business on the court. Some players feel that they are not being good sports if they do not compliment their opponents on good shots. This is simply not the case. It is not at all necessary to compliment opponents on great shots. If your opponent expects to be complimented and doesn't get one, he or she might just think about it a little, which might undermine subsequent performance. You should always act within the rules and show respect for your opponent, but this does not include complimenting him or her on good shots. So if you are the player hitting the great shot, don't expect a compliment from your opponent. If you get one, fine, but if not, just go about the business of playing the match.

Set-Up Points

Brad Gilbert (1993) makes a good point when he discusses points that lead to an ad point (or break point depending on who is serving) which he calls set-up points. Most recreational players tend to consider most points and games in their match as being roughly equivalent with the exception of ad points. Ad points get the blood and adrenaline flowing since players know that a game is on the line, for them, or their opponent. Ad points are noticed. They are obvious and they get special treatment. But the points that lead to ad points (known here as set-up points) are also very important and can bring with it the opportunity for an ad point to hold serve or break serve. For example, if you are serving and the score is 30-love, 30-15, 30-30, or deuce, the next point is a set-up point for you because it offers the opportunity for an ad point, if you win the next point. Conversely, love-30, 15-30, 30-30, and deuce are set-up points for your opponent. If, for example, you are going to break serve, you have to get a break point, and set-up points always precede break points. From a psychological perspective, most club players do not give a lot of weight to set-up points. Their wake-up call is the ad point, not the point preceding it, the set-up point. But your attention should be heightened on set-up points. So how should you play these points.

The first cardinal rule of set-up points (for either you or your opponent) is to get the ball in play whether that means taking a little off your serve and getting it in or making sure your return is in play. It is surprising how often club players will double-fault or carelessly hit a service return out on a set-up point. Most players simply don't understand the importance of set-up points and what they mean to the dynamics of a match. If you're serving at 30-love, for example, understand that if you win that point, you have three consecutive opportunities to win the game. Now is not the time for a double fault or loose shot although many players are not concerned since they still feel they are ahead 30-15. Although that may be the case, you now need to win the next point or else the game is tied at 30-30 and anything can happen. I know that I have lost a lot of games serving at 30-love because I didn't understand the significance of the situation and played a couple of "loose" points.

Once the point is under way, you should hit high percentage shots that do not carry unnecessary risks. Now is not the time to go for the "miracle" shot which you hit one out of ten times. Let your opponent hit the great shot. And if they do, just move on to the next point. But don't give them the point with poor shot selection and decision-making. Finally, try to put the pressure on your opponent at these crucial times. It's always more difficult to hit a passing shot with the pressure on you. And if your opponent is ahead, he or she may be a little lackadaisical and not realize the importance of this set-up point (thus go for a low-percentage shot).

Psychological Momentum

All of you reading this book have probably experienced shifts in momentum in tennis matches. You might have been up 6-2, 4-2 with everything seemingly under control only to have your opponent turn things around (sometimes this appears to hinge on a single point or shot). Sometimes the opposite might have been true, as you turned a match around that you seemed destined to lose. Other times you might have seen dramatic shifts within a match such as winning the first set 6-0 only to lose the second set 0-6. Finally, there are times when these shifts might be even more subtle, and happen numerous times throughout a match. We have traditionally called these changes in momentum, but what really is this thing we call momentum? Of course momentum is extremely difficult to define, as most times it is invisible or at least hard to put your finger on. But usually, momentum is the flow of energy between competitors and thus is related to how we feel and how we think (and often how we play). Why it's often hidden is that momentum does not always follow the score, and the score does not always reflect past momentum. For example, two runners might be tied in a race but one may have the momentum (they may have a great finishing "kick"). Similarly, the score in tennis does not necessarily reflect things such as (a) who is getting tired; (b) who has missed chances; (c) who is just figuring out tactics to win points; (d) who is starting to play better; and (e) who is getting pumped up versus getting discouraged. Table 11.1 gives you some tips on how you know if momentum is with you or against you.

Table 11.1	Is Momentum For or Against You?
Momentum With You	**Momentum Against You**
You feel in control	Nothing seems to be working
The ball and court seem so big	The ball and the court seem so small
Lucky things seem to happen	Unlucky things seem to happen
You move to the ball easily	Your legs feel like lead
You are relaxed but focused	You feel unsettled
Your strokes feel smooth and effortless	Your opponent is controlling play
You don't worry about the score or losing	Small things get on your nerves

It's interesting that a given point may or may not signal a change in momentum—it really depends on how you react to that point and what you do after it that really counts. For example, you might be ahead 6-2, 4-2, 40-30 (serving) and have an easy overhead to win the point and game but you blow it and just miss it wide. Now, this could signal a change in momentum if your opponent seizes the opportunity and wins the next two points and breaks your serve. Or you could simply regroup and win your serve and then serve out the match in your next service game. So if you look at this point after the match, it might be seen as a momentum shift or not, depending on how the players reacted to the point. But when momentum does shift, it usually is tied to some sort of turning point which could include (a) a disputed line call, (b) opponent changing tactics, (c) gamesmanship, (d) missing/making a critical shot, (e) losing a close set, or (f) winning/losing a long game. What turning points have in common is that they have the potential to cause a change in the balance of mental energy of one player or the other, resulting in what we call a change in momentum. But as I noted before, these turning points are only potential turning points. They will end up either as a turning point or merely a blip, depending on your response to the event. So let's look at what you might do if momentum is with you or against you.

Momentum Is With You

When momentum is with you, it appears that there is clear sailing ahead, you are in control, and are confident in your shots. Although this might be the case, you are always very close to having this momentum switched around (especially if your opponent is of similar ability to you), so you have to guard against losing this momentum. You can probably avert this change in momentum if you do follow these tips put forth by Higham (2000).

Stay Focused. A big lead is usually bigger than it seems. A 6-2, 4-1 lead may only be one service break in the second set. It is important that you understand the scoring system because time will not run out on your opponent, like in some other sports. You may seem poised for an easy victory, but the tables can turn quickly if you temporarily become distracted. You don't want to give your opponent the feeling that he or she can win, so stay focused and close out the match.

Stay With What Brought You There. Understand why you are winning and keep up that strategy as you continue through a match. Too many times, players forget why they are winning and revert back to different styles of play, letting their opponents back in the match.

Be Prepared for a Change in Tactics. A player who is losing may very well decide to change her tactics and at least give you something different to look at, whether she slows down the pace of shot, becomes more aggressive rushing the net, or hits out more. Although you may not immediately know the best answer to these different tactics, you should not be surprised by them. Remember that this is your opponent's second choice of tactics, and they probably are not as skilled at it as their first choice. So if you can remain focused and combat this change effectively right away, then your opponent will likely give up these tactics pretty readily.

Be Prepared to Fight. It is easy to let down as you grab what you feel is a commanding lead. But good competitors who get close to losing will usually loosen up and raise the level of their games. So you always have to be ready to scratch and claw for every point and go to battle. Fighting spirit is just as important when you're ahead as when you are behind. So be prepared to fight, even if you don't always have to.

Win the First Point. Although it always makes sense to win the first point of each game, it is especially important at this time because you want to keep your opponent down and believing that he or she cannot win. You want to discourage your opponent and take any sign of hope away. If you win the first point, you won't be facing 0-30 or 0-40 situations, which might energize your opponent.

Momentum Against You

When you perceive that momentum is against you, things can get pretty frustrating. You can't seem to win the important points, you are not really "into the match," you seem unlucky, and you simply aren't playing well. This would seem like enough to "throw in the towel." But good competitors don't give up or give in when faced with these aversive situations. So what can you do when the momentum appears to be against you?

Stay Positive. Probably the most important thing you can do when you feel that everything is going against you is to maintain a positive attitude. This means keeping your thoughts positive (as we discussed in Chapter 9) as well as your body language positive (shoulders back, head up). This will help you keep your energy high and view the match as a challenge to be met, instead of as a disaster.

Closely Monitor Your Tactics. When players feel that the momentum is against them, a typical response is to change tactics. Sometimes this is a good idea as you at least give your opponent something different to look at. But at other times this is a poor decision, since what you were doing was well-thought out; you just were not executing properly. So let's say you wanted to take short balls and hit them aggressively to control the point, but you were either missing your approach shot or simply missing easy volleys. In this case, you might want to continue with your plan. The plan was a good one; you just need to execute better.

Slow Down. When you are losing rapidly and things seem to be going against you, it is easy to rush and speed up play to get off the court (since being on the court is frustrating and anxiety-producing). I mentioned slowing down earlier, and it is especially important when things appear to be spiraling against you. So take your time between serves, let the server wait until you are ready to return (within the rules), and just think about what you need to do to turn things around.

Stay Present Focused. Although this is always a good thing to do, it is especially important when momentum appears to be against you. It is easy to look back at opportunities or shots you missed or look forward to losing the match. But you have to remember the scoring system and sometimes one shot or one game can turn things around. But you have to give yourself a chance for this to happen. So hang in there and try to figure out how best to win the upcoming point. If you win enough points you will find yourself with turning point opportunities.

Being Alert for Patterns of Play. Most players prefer to hit certain shots under certain situations (especially when the pressure is high). For example, they may like to pass cross-court, hit overheads to the open court, serve down the middle, or lob on short balls. If you make a mental note of these propensities, you might be able to guess right at a critical time in the match. Thus, you outguess your opponent and turn her winner into a winner of your own. This can turn things around in a hurry.

Psychology of Doubles

Up to now, I have focused on singles competition (although most of the skills discussed (e.g., imagery, anxiety management, goal-setting, self-talk) could be applied to doubles. But as players grow older, there is more interest in doubles at the recreational levels. This is because of physical limitations (e.g., movement capabilities) and the fact that doubles offers more in the way of a social situation, which many players find attractive. Of course the types of strokes needed for doubles are different from singles with usually more emphasis on the serve and net play. But doubles also differs from singles on the psychological level with more emphasis on interpersonal relationships and communication. This is why some players tend to be more suited for doubles than for singles or why some mediocre (by professional standards) singles players make for a great doubles team (e.g., Mark Woodforde and Todd Woodbridge). Since communication between partners is critical for doubles success, we will focus on the communication process as well as potential problems (and solutions) that might arise in doubles.

Communicating With Your Partner

The key to good doubles play is effective communication between yourself and your partner. But the first step is finding and choosing a partner. From a physical skills perspective, the basic principle to is find someone who will complement your skills. This will help present a balanced attack and adds versatility and flexibility to your doubles game. Thus, if you tend to hit big shots but also make mistakes, it might be a good idea to choose a partner who is steady and makes few unforced errors. This will allow you to be aggressive and go for your shots, since your partner is steady and makes few unforced errors. On the other hand, your partner knows that you can put the ball away so he or she doesn't need to over-hit or take unnecessary chances. From a psychological perspective (and this is probably more important for doubles players over the long haul) it is important to find a partner who you can communicate with well and with whom you enjoy being on the court. Of course you want to play well and be successful, but to stay with a partner requires that you enjoy playing with that person. This doesn't necessarily mean that you have to be good friends off the court. Rather, the key is to harness any differences that might exist between you and your partner, and to work together to produce a stronger psychological unit. Once you've chosen a partner, the next step is effective communication while on the court.

Honesty is the Best Policy

Feedback between two players should be contingent upon performance. Don't compliment someone if they are playing poorly and making bad decisions. Most players know when they are playing poorly, so compliments might just get them annoyed since they know they are not based on their performance. Being honest doesn't mean saying "that was a terrible shot you just hit." But it does mean that you are not afraid to say what you feel if it will be helpful to your partner. Doubles partners also need to be honest in assessing their skills and abilities. If you are uncomfortable hitting overheads, then your partner should know it. Or if you tend to lob off your weaker backhand side, then your partner should know that to get in better position. Don't let your ego get in the way of identifying your strengths and weaknesses. If your second serve is weak, this is important information for your partner.

Besides being honest about your physical capabilities, you also need to be honest about your psychological needs. For example; (a) do you like your partner to be quiet ?; (b) do you need a lot of encouragement?; (c) what should your partner say (if anything) after a bad mistake?; (d) do you like to talk in pressure situations?; (e) do you like to get instructions on what you're doing wrong?; and (f) what helps build your confidence?

Do Not Apologize For Errors

Although you might feel compelled to apologize after making a mistake, this is generally not a good idea in doubles. One reason is that apologizing simply focuses your attention (and your partner's) on the error you just made. You both know you missed an easy overhead, so why bring it up again. A second reason is that apologizing for your errors typically undermines your confidence and builds the confidence of your opponents. Apologizing may just make you feel guilty that you are letting down your partner. Third, apologizing for errors only confirms the fact that you are not playing well. This might even irritate your partner and get him or her thinking about your poor play instead of concentrating on the ball. The best advice is to simply keep quiet after a mistake and immediately focus on the next point.

Support Your Partner

Probably the most important rule to follow in doubles is that you always need to support your partner from an emotional point of view. This requires knowing your partner so you can be supportive, especially when things are not going your way. Talking before matches and finding out what is most helpful for your partner, will help you communicate more effectively in these situations. In a difficult, tight match, it is critical that each player supports his or her partner, so that you both can play to the best of your abilities when the pressure is greatest. This could mean brief statements like "hang in there," "let's get back that break now," or "it's okay, just keep hitting your shots." But knowing what your partner needs and will respond most positively to, is the key to these statements being effective in showing support for your partner. When your partner is playing well, it's also important to show your support (although generally easier than when your partner is playing poorly). So compliment after good shots, which doesn't necessarily mean compliment after every good shot (in this case the compliment loses some of its strength and effectiveness). Therefore, when your partner wins a key point, or hits a really good or smart shot, reinforce that person with statements such as, "great hit," "way to keep your return low," or "great hustle."

Communicate in Preparation for the Next Point

If you watch Davis Cup where there is an emphasis on the critical doubles match, you will see teams constantly meeting after every point (especially when serving). This is not a social meeting but rather a time to communicate what you want to do on the next point. You might very well be deciding where and what kind of serve to hit as well as whether to poach or not. The receiving team may discuss the type of return they will try to hit and whether they will attack the net or not. In any case, it is important to communicate to your partner your intentions before you start the next point, so they can understand and anticipate what you are likely to do. This helps the coordination of the team and frankly is simply more fun.

Build Your Partner's Confidence

In Chapter 5, I discussed the importance of confidence and this certainly applies to the game of doubles. In this case, not only do you have to keep your own confidence up, but you should also try to help keep your partner's confidence high. This is easier said than done, since a missed shot, double fault, blown overhead, or ill-timed drop shot, lets your partner down as well as you. So you might feel especially down after missing an easy shot and this can weigh on your confidence. It's easy to become detached from your partner, especially if you are playing well and your partner is playing poorly. But this is just the time your partner needs your support and encouragement to hang in there. If partners don't show confidence in one another, then their chances of success as a team become greatly diminished.

The difficult thing is to know what to do when your partner is missing easy shots and costing you games. This is where knowing your partner comes in handy. Some people will react positively to a light joke to maybe break the tension. Others need words of encouragement or specific technical instruction. Still others just need their partners to be quiet and not say anything. In essence, the appropriateness of a given response depends on the situation and the personality of your partner. So be supportive but don't get so involved with your partner that you lose your own focus. It's a fine line to balance but one that successful doubles teams do really well.

Keep Talking to a Minimum

Although it most certainly is important to communicate in doubles, don't get the idea that you need to be talking all the time. I have sometimes been in doubles matches where players are talking non-stop because they think it's a social outing (this really drives me crazy and undermines my concentration). When playing competitive tennis, keep your conversations to a minimum and don't really communicate to your opponents. Unless you are out for a social event and everyone agrees to talk throughout the match, you should keep your talking to a minimum, even if you are friends with the players on the court. There will be plenty of time to talk after the match, but stay task-focused during the match. Keep your communication to specific strategy you want to carry out and leave the other conversation for after the match.

Nonverbal Communication

I have been emphasizing verbal communication thus far, but research has clearly revealed the importance of nonverbal communication in conveying information. Some of nonverbal communication is unintentional and thus we are often unaware of the messages we might be sending our partner. Since our nonverbal communication is often unconscious, it more aptly conveys our true feelings. So even if you somehow refrain from making any negative comments to your partner (who is playing really poorly), your nonverbal cues such as slumped shoulders, scowl on your face, and head down would convey your disappointment and possibly disapproval to your partner. Therefore, it is important that you keep aware of your nonverbal cues (in addition to your verbal cues), so that your positive communication matches how you hold yourself and the way you look. This sustains your partner's confidence, and at the same time, lets your opponents know that you are still very much into the match.

Increasing Your Communication Skills

Although I provided a few tips while discussing the process of communication for tennis doubles, let me briefly present some specific ways in which you can improve your communication skills. One thing you could do is try some role-playing, where you take the point of view of the other person (in this case your partner). The goal is to experience what your partner is going through, so that you might change your communication pattern accordingly. For example, let's say that you like to give instruction to your partner when he makes a mistake. In role-playing, you would experience how it feels to receive instruction after every missed shot. Does that bother you or do you become upset? In any case you would experience how it feels from your partner's point of view, which should give you a better understanding of your partner's thoughts and feelings.

Another tool to raise the consciousness of our communication patterns is to keep a *logbook*. This type of self-monitoring helps you keep track of what you say and when you say it, which is usually the first step to making any kind of behavior change. So after you play some doubles, ask yourself a few questions and record your answers in your log. For example, you might ask yourself, "Was I positive today?" "What did I say after my partner made a mistake?" "Did I use any criticism?" "Did I communicate poorly in any situations?" or "What did I communicate non-verbally?"

A final method to help improve your communication is again through the use of imagery. Using the principles of imagery discussed in Chapter 7, you could visualize particular situations and see yourself communicating in a positive manner that would help both of you. For example, let's say you often start to get angry and negative when your partner repeatedly misses relatively easy shots. In your imagery, you could create these same situations and then see yourself being positive and supportive and your partner reacting with an improvement in his play.

CHAPTER 12

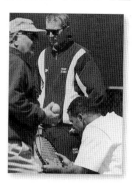

PARENTS AND YOUNG TENNIS PLAYERS

There is no doubt that parents exert a tremendous effect on their tennis playing sons and daughters. We can look at today's professional players and find many examples of parents who had a negative or positive influence on their tennis-playing child and teenager (and sometimes adult). But there are far more parents of young tennis players who never make it to the pros who need some direction and guidelines for bringing up a young tennis player. As Chris Evert has noted:

> *When I was growing up and playing junior tennis in the 1960's, my mother would drive me and my brother and sisters and maybe some other kids from our tennis park to a tournament. Afterwards, we'd all go to the mall or have pizza together. That was life in the juniors.... Today's emphasis on money has introduced some very negative elements into the game of tennis, not the least of which is the often outrageous behavior of parents at junior tournaments.*
>
> *(USA Tennis Parents Guide, p. vii)*

Although this may be an oversimplification, raising a young tennis player is certainly more complicated today. In fact, in my tennis workshops and consultations as well as talking to colleagues at the United States Tennis Association, it is obvious that parents need help in knowing how best to work with their young tennis-playing children. Parents themselves, are seeking out additional information, trying to find the best way to raise their tennis-playing child. Therefore, this chapter will be dedicated to providing parents with the latest scientific information (particularly, psychological and developmental) to help produce the most positive tennis experience for their children.

Keeping Winning in Perspective

Probably more than anything else, parents need to help their children keep winning in perspective. This does not mean that winning is unimportant; rather it means that winning is simply not the sole focus when a player goes out on the court. A good place to start in terms of where winning fits in for young tennis players, is the many studies conducted on why children want to play in competitive sports. Across sports, the most consistent reasons for children's participation were to *have fun, to learn skills,* and to *be with friends.* Winning usually ranks down on the list and is virtually never given as one of the top three reasons.

Probably the greatest error parents can make is to voice expectations for their child beyond simply having a good time and enjoying the experience. Unfortunately, after a tennis match, most young players hear the following from their parents, "Did you win?" Instead, parents could simply ask their children, "How did you play?" or "Did you have fun today?" Even on disastrous days, something positive could be said such as, "I guess you didn't play that well today, but I liked the way you kept trying." As soon as a child starts playing for parental approval or to maintain harmony in the family, the player's motivation will inevitably diminish, regardless of his or her level of talent. Many young players with potential have been turned off to tennis by their parents, and some great talents have been destroyed in this fashion. Think of all the pressure a young tennis player must feel, when playing for the love and approval of a parent. Now that's pressure.

Parental pressure can take many forms including: (a) forcing the child to take lessons, practice, or compete in matches against his or her will; (b) constant criticism of the child's efforts; (c) constant overbearing behavior at matches and practices; (d) holding how much financial investment was made in the player over his or her head; and (e) expectations of high achievement—not accepting defeat. None of these will typically have long-term effects if they happen only once or twice. However, constantly putting pressure on a child will inevitably be disastrous. Sometimes this pressure is not even intentional. For example, I worked with a teenage player who said that every time he was playing poorly and needed emotional support, he would look to his father who would simply shake his head in disgust. This can utterly destroy a young player's confidence and belief in his abilities. When asked about this, his father said, "I did not even realize that I was giving off such a negative signal." (note that the father stopped this behavior when he was made aware of it and the negative influence it had on his child). Of course this is more subtle than parents who constantly put down and criticize their child, force them to practice every day, or make unflattering comparisons with other tennis-playing kids. But it's really the child's perception that is critical and parents, therefore, need to make sure the experience is a fun and enjoyable one, not a pressure-filled one.

One of the ways to make things more fun and downplay winning is to have your child focus on achieving performance goals, rather than outcome goals (discussed in detail in Chapter 4). Performance goals are more under the control of the player and can help improve his or her game whereas outcome (winning/losing) goals are out of a player's control since they depend in large part on how well your opponent plays. For example, as noted earlier, when Pete Sampras and his coach decided to change from a two-handed to one-handed backhand, they knew that the short-term outcomes would be poorer. But it was their belief that Sampras' performance would be better and more improved over the long run if the change was made (they were certainly right). Unfortunately, too many junior players (and their parents) opt to keep the focus on winning, rather than long-term development. This might result in more wins (outcome goal) in the short-term, but there is not going to be as much improvement (performance goal) over the long-term. That is one reason why I am against all the many rankings (e.g., district, state, regional, national) that prevail at the junior level. This often has the unfortunate result of focusing players' and parents' attention on rankings (won-loss records) rather than on improving one's game. You can often win in the juniors by simply getting the ball back and playing safe. But that usually won't be good enough as players get older and need more shots in their arsenal. So, use the principles put forth in Chapter 4 and set performance-oriented goals, both in practices and matches. This will not only help you improve, but it should also eventually help you be more successful in the future. Most of all, remember to keep things fun, because this is the primary reason that kids choose to play competitive sport in the first place.

Conducting Yourself as a Tennis Parent

I am often asked by tennis parents for some suggestions regarding proper conduct and etiquette. Of course you basically want to follow good common sense and be supportive of your child. One key thing, though, is to make sure you are a good role model (and choose a coach who is also a good role model). This means (among other things) that you don't yell and scream at the officials, get into a heated argument with another parent, or yell at your kid when he or she hits a bad shot. But there are several guidelines to follow to make your behavior even more positive, both on and off the court, and these are displayed in Table 12.1. Included in Table 12.1 are also some of your basic responsibilities as a tennis parent.

Making Good Decisions

As a tennis parent (or any parent for that matter), we have to make many decisions regarding the well-being and welfare of our children. These decisions are not always easy and there are many typical ones that tennis-parents have to come to grips with at one point or another. Some of the tough questions that tennis-parents face that eventually may require some decision-making include: (a) Shouldn't I be upset if my son plays badly and doesn't even appear to try? (b) My daughter wants to quit tennis after I spent so much money on lessons, camps, and pros. Should I just let her quit? (c) Is it normal for a kid to get injured so much? (d) I saw my son call good shots out during a match. Should I say something to him or the tournament director? (e) At what age should my daughter start to play competitive tennis? and (f) I know my son has some talent but he just doesn't want to train hard. Should I push him? I will try to provide some guidelines (see Loehr & Smith, 2001 for a more detailed discussion) for answering these questions and questions like these.

Table 12.1	Positive Behaviors and Responsibilities for Tennis Parents

Show enthusiasm, interest and support of your child

Don't tell the coach how to do his (her) job

Keep control of your emotions

Do not insult opposing players, coaches, parents, or officials

Help when asked to be an official or coach

Do not try to coach your child

Remain in the spectator area during competitions

Understand why your child plays tennis and provide reinforcement for this goal

Keep perspective and balance–tennis should be just one part of the child's life

Discipline your child when necessary –being a good sport is important

Encourage but do not pressure your child to play tennis

Help your child understand responsibilities to the team and coach

Find a qualified coach or teaching pro to help guide your child.

Provide reinforcement regardless of match outcome and performance

Note: Adapted from Lubbers (2001) Keeping Your Child's Tennis in Perspective (p. 8) *USA Tennis Parents' Guide.*

Make Decisions Based Upon Your Child as a Person, Not a Player

The primary role of parents is to make sure that the tennis experience has a positive impact on the long-term health and happiness of their child. There is a fine line between encouraging and supporting your child and pushing him or her too hard. The real measure of success in tennis, is the impact it has on your child's long-term health and happiness. The primary role of a parent is to love and care for a child, no matter what he or she chooses to do in life. As noted earlier, sometimes parents send messages to children that their love is somehow contingent on how well the child plays on the tennis court. Whether intentional or not, the child needs to know that the parents love him or her regardless of any outcome on the tennis court. So make sure that you make decisions in the best interest of your child as a person, and not simply what happens to be better for his or her tennis career.

Make Decisions to Enhance Enjoyment and Reduce the Probability of Burnout

Research by Gould, Tuffy, Udry, and Loehr (1997) has clearly indicated that burnout in young tennis players occurs primarily due to both psychological and physiological reasons.

From a physical standpoint, make sure your tennis-playing child eats, sleeps, and drinks properly as noted in Chapter 10. In addition, you want to avoid overtraining, that is, putting too many hours on the tennis court on a day-to-day basis as well as constantly talking about tennis off the court. Along these lines, you should consider having your child participate in other sports (e.g., soccer, basketball) when they are young, as this not only can enhance the fun aspect of competitive sports, but also can build skills important for tennis such as movement, balance, and coordination. The team aspect of these other sports can also help provide for the need for affiliation, so important to youngsters.

This does not mean avoiding tournaments or other types of competition. But tournaments can be made more fun, for example, by taking some time away from the court and joining your child (maybe bring along some of his or her friends) in other activities such as going to the mall, playing miniature golf, going to see a movie, playing video games, or going for a boat ride. These off-the-court experiences are sometimes the highlight of the weekend—remember the importance of fun and affiliation motives for young tennis players.

The second aspect of burnout is more psychological in nature and revolves around the perfectionist attitude of the players, as well as the critical nature of many parents and coaches. Because some young players are perfectionism-oriented based on their personalities, they are usually very hard on themselves in the first place. These types of young tennis players do not need coaches and parents to get on their case and be very critical of their play. They are already very critical of themselves (too critical) in an attempt to be perfect (which of course nobody is perfect). So support, encouragement, and positive feedback should be provided as much as possible to help make tennis an enjoyable experience, one in which the child will want to continue for the rest of his or her life.

Make Decisions Based on Your Child's Best Interests, Not Your Own

Before you make important decisions regarding the role of tennis in your child's life, make sure you remember to make the decision based on your child's needs and interests and not your own. You have to make sure that you are not using the child's success in tennis to meet some unfulfilled need that you might have for success and recognition. It is certainly easy to get wrapped up in your child's tennis and this happens all too often. Some parents simply try to meet their own aspirations through their kids and this can only lead to disaster. So take a step back when making decisions and make sure you have the best interests of your child in mind, not your own best interests.

Make Decisions That Foster the Psychosocial Development of Your Child

One of the key questions parents can ask themselves is, "Do I like the person my child is becoming because of tennis?" Like other sports, tennis can be a great avenue to learn psychological, social, and moral skills, but it does not happen automatically. Some players really develop as tennis players, but lag behind as people. For example, as noted earlier, one of the things that distinguishes tennis from most other sports, is that players act as their own referees in calling lines and keeping score. This is a very difficult and challenging task, to say the least. Unfortunately, if you are a tennis parent, it is almost inevitable that some players at tournaments are known to "cheat" on line calls or at least not be very fair in their calls. Parents must insist that their children call lines fairly and not resort to cheating to win matches. Many kids who cheat, do so (at least in part) because of the pressure put on them to win by parents. Young tennis players should be reinforced for being fair and giving their opponent the benefit of the doubt on close calls that they cannot see clearly. The highest measures of success should always be honesty, sportsmanship, personal ethics, and respect for one's opponent. These are the characteristics parents should want to have their child learn from tennis and keep with them through a lifetime.

Make Decisions (Goals) Based on Performance, Not Outcome

Probably most parents who have a young, talented (at least they believe to be talented) tennis player, hope that they might be a touring professional some day, or at least get a college scholarship for tennis. Although this might happen (but the odds are very much against it—especially becoming a professional), the goal that should be pursued is continued improvement and personal development. As noted by Loehr and Smith (2001, p. 13), "If all the sacrifices, time, and money invested can only be justified if your child becomes a successful touring professional, you're on a collision course with disaster." The time and money you invest in your child's tennis playing career, should be seen as an investment in his or her development as a person. If they happen to be successful in tennis, then that's great, but that should not be the end goal.

Developmental Considerations

As a tennis parent, it is important that you know and appreciate the different developmental stages that your child may go through so that you can provide helpful guidance and assistance, appropriate to the developmental level of your child. Sometimes, parents get frustrated with a lack of improvement or development and this may be just typical of the age of your child. As the mental health professionals say, it may be age-appropriate behavior. It is beyond the scope of the book to provide an in-depth analysis of developmental stages that children go through. Rather I will try to highlight some of the key issues for tennis parents, so they better understand the growth and development of their child (see Woods, 2001 for a more complete discussion). Before, these are discussed, four basic principles of child development should be kept in mind.

- Stages of growth are determined more by physiological age, rather than chronological age. Some children mature early, and some mature late from a physical point of view. Each child is different and goes though these stages differently.

- Consider development and maturation of children from different perspectives, including physical, social, mental, and emotional.
- Children are not miniature adults and should not be treated as such. Youth sport coaches often forget this principle and treat young players like professionals and are disappointed when they just act like "kids."
- Children rely a lot on role models. So make sure as a parent you are a good role model. If you lose your temper on the sidelines, you can't expect your youngster to remain cool and calm at all times.

Ages 4-7

At this early age, children are typically just learning basic motor activities such as jumping, running, twisting and turning, as well as some basic hand-eye coordination. Parents and coaches should keep things very simple and try to demonstrate tasks and skills to be learned, rather than giving extended verbal instructions. Children tend to be very inquisitive, so help them learn by asking questions and setting up situations for them to explore. Tennis instruction should focus on having fun although some basic tennis techniques can be acquired. Too much emphasis on skill refinement at this age is not warranted, since children have not yet developed the fine motor control necessary, and their attention spans are generally too short. So keep it *fun* and *simple*.

Ages 8-11

The key point here is that it is still too early to start to specialize in tennis. Provide children with a wide array of movement activities so they can improve their overall motor development. Parents still have a big influence on their kids as they typically want to follow the rules and win the approval of significant others. There are wide ranges in physical abilities as some children start to mature earlier than others. So, some players might be more successful than others at an early age simply because they have matured earlier. Expectations, therefore, for these kids are often high, but yet their success now is not based on physical skills, rather it is just quicker development and others will catch up in the ensuing years. Also, don't forget the later maturing child who may not be successful early based on their later development. Don't give up on this child as they may blossom over the next few years. Remember that Michael Jordan was cut from his high school team and he turned out pretty well!

In terms of tennis itself, the focus should be on the "game of tennis" rather than simply honing down individual strokes. Children at this age should try to understand how the shots fit together within a game situation. Fundamental skills need to be taught but then experimented with in game situations. To protect against injury (especially since the skeletal system is still developing), strength training, primarily using the player's own body weight (e.g., sit-ups, push-ups) should be employed, as well as flexibility training to increase range of movement.

Ages 12-15

This is an age period characterized by rapid growth and change for both boys and girls. But boys and girls will also mature differently during this time as puberty usually occurs . In large part due to the onset of puberty, girls will typically mature earlier and faster than boys with girls experiencing their growth spurt two years earlier than boys. These differences in the onset of puberty usually lead to wide variations in height and weight of kids of the same chronological age, leading to self-consciousness and confidence issues. At this time there is sometimes even a regression in skills as the young tennis player is getting used to a body that is changing very rapidly.

There is a definite change in mental development, as the early adolescent can better start to understand sportspersonship and its importance. Social development is strongly affected by peer groups and young teens try to be part of a group. Self-worth and tennis performance often get confused at this stage (especially if the parents and coaches are not vigilant in stressing effort and improvement over results and rankings). Outcome of matches are often determined by maturation rates, rather than tennis ability (as these differ widely among players), which is another reason to focus on process and performance goals. Finally, this is a time when the foundation of strokes and skills are honed and will typically change little over the years. Therefore, it's a good time to experiment with different playing styles, selecting one that works best for the player and that is fun to play.

Ages 16-18

This is an age when girls typically start to plateau based on their early growth spurt and thus they can easily become discouraged and frustrated with their rate of progress in improving their tennis game. Boys, on the other hand, will typically experience continued improvement due to their later growth spurt and thus their enthusiasm and commitment is more likely to remain high. Like any other teenager of this age, there is a questioning of authority and their thought processes are typically more advanced than their social and emotional skills. The peer group continues to be extremely important although there is a move toward more independence which parents should reinforce, if they want to assist the transition to a responsible adult. Of course decisions about college start to become more important (as well as decisions about dating, jobs, and driving) and parents should be involved, interested, and supportive. At this time, most players come to realize that they won't become professional players, but rather they should focus on rounding out their games in order to compete successfully in high school or college. Players should be encouraged to adopt a style of play that best suits them, as well as starting (or continuing) to develop the mental skills necessary to be successful in a competitive tennis environment.

Choosing a Coach/Teaching Pro

Thus far, I have focused mostly on what parents should do, especially their behavior toward their young tennis-playing children. But one of the key parts of being a parent is helping a child choose a coach that fits his or her interests, needs, and abilities. I noted earlier that generally speaking, a parent should not coach his or her child (unless they have specific tennis skills and background as well as understanding the emotional and psychological part of coaching his or her own child). There are some examples such as Martina Hingis and the Williams sisters who were coached by their parent(s) but in general this is a difficult ball to juggle. In most cases, a parent needs to find the right coach or teaching pro who will maximize the child's potential and create a positive and productive experience for him or her. Table 12.2 provides a summary of some of the key attributes that should be considered by parents when choosing a coach/teaching pro.

Parents should stay in close contact with coaches although they should not interfere with the day-to-day lessons and practices of coaches. They most certainly should get feedback from coaches concerning the progress of their child as well as explanations for why certain approaches are taken. Questions could and should be asked to learn more about the style of the coach. The parents hire the coach but that doesn't give them the right to interfere with the coach. Of course it's the parents' right to evaluate the coaches on the items listed in Table 12.2. And if a coaching change is called for, then the parents (in discussion with the player –especially if the player is old enough to provide useful input) should look for a different coach. But this should be done in a thoughtful, deliberate manner, getting feedback from all relevant parties, before a change is made. Remember, that if parents choose a coach wisely (using the criteria listed in Table 12.2), then there will probably not be a need to change coaches (or at least the need would be less likely). The United States Tennis Association has published a guide to help parents' of young tennis players and that provides more detailed suggestions for parents in helping their young tennis playing child. (*USA Tennis Parents' Guide*).

Table 12.2	Skills and Behaviors of Good Coaches/Teachers
Characteristic	**Specific Behavior(s)**
Communication	• Focuses on positive instead of negative • Instructions are clear and concise • Instructions are contingent on behavior • Listens carefully and effectively
Knowledge	• Knows how to teach tennis skills • Knowledgeable about tactics and strategy • Knowledgeable about sport sciences such as sport psychology, physiology, and medicine • Knowledge about training and drilling and learning progressions
Coaching Philosophy	• Emphasizes skill development and enjoyment • Keeps winning and losing in perspective • Focuses on process and improvement, not outcome
Self-Control	• Displays self-control on and off the court • Provides a good role model for the player • Maintains composure even when players make mistakes and errors
Enthusiasm	• Is enthusiastic about playing and coaching • Helps build enthusiasm in players
Understanding	• Understands developmental differences among players and treats them accordingly • Understands that mistakes are part of learning Maintains a consistent approach - not hypo-critical

Note: Adapted from Saviano (2001) The role of tennis coaches (p. 27)
USA Tennis Parents' Guide.

References

Baumeister, R., & Steinhilber, A. (1984). Paradoxical effects of supportive audiences on performance under pressure: The home field disadvantage in sports championships. *Journal of Personality and Social Psychology, 43,* 85-93.

Bell, K. (1983). *Championship thinking.* Englewood Cliffs, NJ: Prentice Hall.

Benson, H., & Proctor, W. (1984). *Beyond the relaxation response.* New York: Berkley.

Butler, R., & Hardy, L. (1992). The performance profile: Theory and application. *The Sport Psychologist, 6,*253-264.

Eisenman, P., Johnson, S., & Benson, J. (1990). *Coaches guide to nutrition and weight control.* (2nd ed.). Champaign, IL: Human Kinetics.

Ellis, A. (1962). *Reason and emotion in psychotherapy.* New York: Lyle Stuart.

Filby, W.C.D., Maynard, I.W., & Graydon, J.K. (1999). The effect of multiple-goal strategies on performance outcomes in training and competition. *Journal of Applied Sport Psychology, 11,* 230-246.

Fox, A., & Evan, R. (1979). *If I'm the better player, why can't I win.* New York: Tennis Magazine.

Fox, A. (1993). *Think to win: The strategic dimension of tennis.* Harper Collins: New York

Gallwey, T. (1974). *Inner game of tennis.* New York: Random House.

Gilbert, B., & Jamison, S. (1993). *Winning ugly: Mental warfare in tennis—lessons from a master.* Simon & Schuster: New York.

Gould, D., Eklund, R., & Jackson, S. (1992). Coping strategies used by more versus less successful Olympic wrestlers. *Research Quarterly for Exercise and Sport. 64,* 83-93.

Gould, D., Guinan, D., Greenleaf, C., Medbery, R., & Peterson, K. (1999). Factors affecting Olympic performance: Perceptions of athletes and coaches from more and less successful teams. *The Sport Psychologist, 13,* 371-394.

Gould, D., Hodge, K., Peterson, K., & Giannini, J. (1989). An exploratory examination of strategies used by elite coaches to enhance self-efficacy. *Journal of Sport & Exercise Psychology, 11,* 128-140.

Gould, D., Medbery, R., Damarjian, N., & Lauer, L. (1999). A survey of mental skills, training, knowledge, opinions, and practices of junior tennis coaches. *Journal of Applied Sport Psychology,*11, 28-50.

Gould, D., Tuffey, S., Udry, E., & Loehr, J. (1997). Burnout in competitive junior tennis players: III. Individual difference in the burnout experience. *The Sport Psychologist, 11,* 257-276.

Greenleaf, C., Gould, D., & Diffenbach, K. (2001). Factors influencing Olympic performance: Interviews with Atlanta and Nagano U.S. Olympians. *Journal of Applied Sport Psychology, 13,* 154-184.

Hanin, Y. (1997). Emotions and athletic performance: Individual zones of optimal functioning. *European yearbook of sport psychology, 1,* 29-72.

Hardy, L., Gammage, K., & Hall, C. (2001). A descriptive study of athletes' self-talk. *The Sport Psychologist*, 15, 306-318.

Hardy, L., Jones, G., & Gould, D. (1996). *Understanding psychological preparation for sport: Theory and practice for elite performers.* Chichester, England: Wiley.

Higham, A. (2000). *Momentum: The hidden force in tennis.* Leeds, England: 1st 4sport Publications.

Hume, K., Martin, G., Gonzalez, P., Kracklen, C., & Genthon, S. (1985). A self-monitoring package for improving freestyle figure skating practice. *Journal of Sport Psychology*, 7, 333-345.

Ievleva, L., & Orlick, T. (1991). Mental links to enhanced healing. *The Sport Psychologist*, 5, 25-40.

Jacobsen, E. (1938). *Progressive relaxation.* Chicago: University of Chicago Press.

Jackson, S., & Csikszentimalyi, M. (1999). *Flow in sports: The keys to optimal experiences and performances.* Champaign, IL: Human Kinetics.

Jones, G., Hanton, S., & Connaughton, D. (2002). What is mental toughness. *Journal of Applied Sport Psychology*, 14.

Jones, G., & Swain, A. (1995). Predisposition to experience debilitative and facilitative anxiety in elite and non-elite performers. *The Sport Psychologist*, 9, 201-211.

Jones. G., Swain, A., & Hardy, (1993), Intensity and direction dimensions of competitive state anxiety and relationships with performance. *Journal of Sport Sciences*, 11, 525-532.

Kingston, K., & Hardy, L. (1997). Effects of different types of goals on processes that support performance. *The Sport Psychologist*, 11, 277-293.

Kirschenbaum, D. (1997) *Mind matters: Seven steps to smarter sport performance.* Carmel, IN: Cooper.

Locke, L., & Latham, G. (1990). *A theory of goal setting and task performance.* Englewood Cliffs, NJ: Prentice Hall.

Loehr, J., & Smith S. (2001). Helping parents make good decisions. In *USA Tennis Parents' Guide* (pp. 10-15). White Plains, NY: United States Tennis Association.

Phillips, B. (1980, June).The tennis machine, *Time*, 48-58.

Ransom, K., & Weinberg, R. (1985). Effect of situation criticality on the performance of elite male and female tennis players. *Journal of Sport Behavior*, 8, 144-148.

Slaikeu, K., & Trogolo, R. (1998). *Focused on tennis.* Champaign, IL: Human Kinetics

Tarshis, B. (1977). *Tennis and the mind.* New York: Tennis Magazine.

Theodorakis, Y.,Weinberg, R., Natsis P., Douma, I., & Kazakas, P. (2000) The effects of motivational versus instructional self-talk on improving motor performance, *The Sport Psychologist*, 14, 253-272.

USA Tennis Parents' Guide. Key Biscayne, FL: United States Tennis Association.

Van Raalte, J., Brewer, B., Rivera, P., & Petitpas, A. (1994). The relationship between self-talk and performance of competitive junior tennis players. *Journal of Sport & Exercise Psychology*, 16, 400-415.

Vealey, R. (2001). Understanding and enhancing self-confidence in athletes. In R. Singer, H.Hausenblaus, & C. Janelle (Eds.), *Handbook of sport psychology*, 2nd ed. (pp. 550-565). New York: John Wiley and Sons.

Weinberg, R. (1988). *The Mental Advantage: Developing your psychological skills in tennis.* Champaign, IL: Human Kinetics.

Weinberg, R. Burke, K., & Jackson, A. (1997). Coaches and players' perception of goal setting in junior tennis: An exploratory investigation. *The Sport Psychologist,* 11, 426-439.

Weinberg, R., Burton, D., Yukelson, D., & Weigand, D. (1993). Goal setting in competitive sport: An exploratory investigation of practices of collegiate athletes. *The Sport Psychologist,* 7, 275-289.

Weinberg, R., Burton, D., Yukelson, D., & Weigand, D. (2000). Perceived goal setting practices of Olympic athletes: An exploratory investigation. *The Sport Psychologist,* 14, 280-296.

Weinberg, R., Butt, J., & Knight, B. (2001). High school coaches' perceptions of the process of goal setting. *The Sport Psychologist,* 15, 20-47.

Weinberg, R., Butt, J., Knight, B., & Burke, K. (2003). The relationship between the use and effectiveness of imagery: An exploratory study. *Journal of Applied Sport Psychology,* 15.

Weinberg, R., Butt, J., Knight, B., & Perritt, N. (2001). Collegiate coaches' perceptions of their goal-setting practices: A qualitative investigation. *Journal of Applied Sport Psychology,* 13, 374-398.

Weinberg, R., & Gould, D. (1999). *Foundations of sport and exercise psychology.* Champaign, IL: Human Kinetics.

Weinberg, R., Grove, J.R., & Jackson, A. (1992). Strategies for building self-efficacy in tennis players: A comparative analysis of American and Australian coaches. *The Sport Psychologist,* 6, 3-13.

Weinberg, R., & Jackson, A. (1990). Building self-efficacy in tennis players: A coaches' perspective. *Journal of Applied Sport Psychology,* 2, 161-171.

Woods, R. (2001). Child development: Its impact on the young tennis player. In *USA Tennis Parents' Guide* (pp. 16-22). White Plains, NY: United States Tennis Association.

INDEX

INDEX **183**

Ivanisevic, Goran, 7, 11, 60

J

Jackson, A., 44, 57, 65
Jackson, S., 13-14, 113, 120
Jacobson, Edmund, 83
Johnson, Michael, 108
Johnson, S., 148
Jones, G., 22, 89, 126
Jordan, Michael, 16, 27-28

K

Kafelnikov, Yevgeny, 7, 56
Kazakas, P., 130
King, Billie Jean, v, 51, 60
Kingston, K., 37
Kirschenbaum, D., 37, 114
Knight, B., 44, 105
Krackley, C., 124
Kramer, Jack, 140
Kuerten, Gustavo, 6, 58

L

Latham, G., 38
Lauer, L., 5
Laver, Rod, 10-11, 20, 54, 92, 110, 121, 158
Lendl, Ivan, 11-12, 68, 92, 159
Locke, E., 38
Loehr, J., 13, 85, 170-171, 173
Lubbers, P., 171

M

Martens, R., 95
Martin, G., 124
Match play
  mind games and, 153-155
  momentum and, 160-164
  set-up points and, 160
Match preparation

eating/drinking, 148-149
equipment, 148
game plan, 141-144
imagery, 150-151
importance of, 140
routines and, 144-147
stretching, 149-150
warm-up, 151-152
Maynard, I., 38
McEnroe, John, 12, 54, 92, 114, 138, 159
Medbery, R., 5, 7
Mental skills
  assessment, 21-25
  importance of, 1-5
  relationship to body, 3-4
  teaching, 7-9
  time practicing, 6-9
Motivation. see goal-setting

N

Natsis, P., 130
Navratilova, Martina, 4, 25, 68
Newcombe, John, 91, 158
Novotna, Jana, 115

O

Orick, T., 107
Orantes, Manual, 56

P

Parents
  choosing a coach, 176-177
  conducting yourself, 170-173
  developmental considerations, 173-175
  keeping winning in perspective, 169-170
  making good decisions, 170-173
Peak performance. see psychological states
Perritt, N., 44
Peterson, K., 7, 65
Petitpas, A., 130